The Myth of Senility

The Myth of Senility

THE TRUTH ABOUT THE BRAIN AND AGING

Robin Marantz Henig

Foreword by
Robert N. Butler, M.D.

An AARP Book
published by
American Association of Retired Persons
Washington, D.C.
Scott, Foresman and Company
Lifelong Learning Division
Glenview, Illinois

Library of Congress Cataloging-in-Publication Data

Henig, Robin Marantz.
  The myth of senility.

  Bibliography: p.
  Includes index.
  1. Senile dementia.   2. Brain—Aging.   3. Aging.
  4. Alzheimer's disease.   I. Title. [DNLM: 1. Aging.
  2. Dementia, Presenile.   3. Dementia, Senile.
  WT 150 H511m]
  RC524.H46   1985   618.97′688983   85-18369
  ISBN 0-673-24831-3 (Scott, Foresman)

Paperback revised edition published 1985 by Scott, Foresman and Company, Glenview, Illinois, and the American Association of Retired Persons, Washington, D.C.

Originally published in 1981 under the title *The Myth of Senility: Misconceptions About the Brain and Aging* by Anchor Press/Doubleday.

12345678-KPF-91908988878685

AARP Books is an educational and public service project of the American Association of Retired Persons, which, with a membership of 20 million, is the largest association of persons fifty and over in the world today. Founded in 1958, AARP provides older Americans with a wide range of membership programs and services, including legislative representation at both federal and state levels. For further information about additional association activities, write to AARP, 1909 K Street, NW, Washington, DC 20049.

Dedicated in loving memory to my grandparents,
Joseph and Yetta Stern

Contents

Foreword

I have often stated my concern that the term "senility" is overused and little understood. In no other area of medicine is such a nebulous term offered and accepted as a diagnosis. "Senility" is descriptive of a plethora of insults that occur anywhere in the body and cause the confusion, the serious memory lapses, and the deterioration of personality and intellect that are routinely dismissed as inevitable in old age. Because mental impairment can mask more than a hundred different physical and emotional problems in older patients, the symptoms of "senility" should be treated as a medical emergency necessitating comprehensive and sensitive medical diagnosis and care.

"Senility" results in an untold emotional and financial drain on its victims, their families, and society at large. For this reason, the National Institute on Aging developed a concise authoritative statement on the diagnosis of confusion and mental impairment in the elderly, a statement that has been widely circulated to medical professionals. *The Myth of Senility* helps disseminate information on the medical diagnosis of "senility" in a most effective way—by putting knowledge into the hands of people who are taking increasing responsibility for their own health care.

That "senility" is not inevitable in old age is not news to the medical and scientific communities. Since the middle of this century, science and technology have begun to wear away the stereotypes that were responsible for much professional disinterest in the aged. What is new is that geriatric patients are beginning to ask the right questions and demand proper care. Those responsible for health care policy are beginning to recognize the need for training in geriatrics in U.S. medical schools in the context of an elderly population that will double by the year 2030, reaching 55 million persons. Professional medical societies, private organizations, and a number of government agencies have taken a stand on the need to promote geriatric medicine and clinical research on aging. Medical students and young physicians have been particularly adamant in seeking information on the appropriate care and management of elderly patients. They are also seeking the answers that only scientific research can provide. After all, physicians of the not so distant future will be spending half of their practice time caring for the elderly.

For as many as 3 million elderly Americans, "senility" is no myth. Alzheimer's disease, the most common form of what is popularly called "senility," is characterized by progressive irreversible intellectual impairment, and is associated with protracted dependency and, ultimately, with death. Alzheimer's disease results in a disproportionately large share of the country's $28 billion expenditure for long-term care. Unless science can pinpoint the cause or causes of Alzheimer's disease, we will have no choice but to continue with the halfway measures of care we now provide, and the costs of ineffective treatment will continue to mount.

Federally sponsored scientific research on Alzheimer's disease has increased by more than 800 percent since the creation of the National Institute on Aging as part of the National Institutes of Health. Scientists are now pursuing many leading theories as to what causes Alzheimer's disease. These theories are as diverse as the disciplines of the experts exploring them—including neurochemistry, toxicology, immunology, genetics, and virology—and Robin Henig will explore them in the chapters to follow. The work comes in the context of scientific achievements of the past few decades: (1) findings that began to separate normal brain aging from age-related disease in the brain; (2) findings that linked the symptoms of dementia with specific pathological changes in the brain; (3) technology that has revolutionized our ability to study brain structure and function and to diagnose disease in its earliest stages; and finally, (4) ongoing studies to develop a clearer understanding of normal brain function and what happens to the brains of Alzheimer's victims.

Other studies will determine if there is a population "at risk" of developing Alzheimer's disease. We know of no link between Alzheimer's and sex, race, occupation, or place of residence, although the disorder, or at least one form of the disorder, does seem to cluster in families. We do know that classic Alzheimer's disease can strike as early as age forty, and that wherever there are old people there is Alzheimer's disease.

The number of people affected also remains unknown. Many escape medical attention by remaining in their home communities because a caring and supportive network compensates for their loss. Others are misdiagnosed. With all the promise of research on the causes of Alzheimer's disease, the diagnosis is still one of exclusion. No single test will definitively identify a patient with Alzheimer's.

Since the advent of deinstitutionalization, fewer and fewer senile dementia cases are being treated in mental institutions. Because of their special needs, they are often rejected by general hospitals and other "mainstream" institutions. As a result, most are concentrated in nursing homes, where they are generally unable to benefit from clinical research programs and the intellectual interest generated in an academic environment. If a patient is young and physically healthy, he or she may even be rejected by most nursing homes. While I personally support the concept of liberalizing home care and giving families the assistance they need to care for patients at home, I believe that the major objective of the health community should be to treat, ameliorate, cure, and ultimately prevent Alzheimer's disease—not simply to shift patients around among mental institutions, nursing homes, or private homes.

Even with the voluminous gaps in our knowledge of how to conquer senile dementia, the picture is not gloomy. Directions and possibilities for future studies are better defined than ever. Interest in geriatric medicine is growing, as is the number of medical schools now sponsoring or planning courses in geriatrics. Public awareness of senile dementia as a pervasive problem has increased, and interest in the newest scientific and medical developments is insatiable. *The Myth of Senility* is a product of this interest and goes a long way toward fulfilling the demands of a broad audience.

Robert N. Butler, M.D.
Brookdale Professor and Chairman,
Ritter Department of Geriatrics and Adult
   Development
Mount Sinai Medical Center
New York, New York

Former Director, National Institute on Aging

Preface

Five years have passed since I wrote *The Myth of Senility,* five years in which knowledge about the aging brain has fairly exploded. When I was researching the book in 1980, my friends thought I was writing about "Old Timers' disease"; now Alzheimer's disease has been designated the disease of the century, and most people know not only how to pronounce it but how to define it.

Indeed, the term "Alzheimer's disease" has become so popular, among both physicians and the public at large, that it is in danger of becoming what the term "senility" has been for a generation: a wastebasket diagnosis into which are heaped all older people who seem to be losing their memories. And that is why there is still a need for this book.

We have come far in five years, but we have not come far enough. Educated, informed people still believe that at least some significant decline in mental functioning is inevitable in old age. Educated, informed people still fear "senility"—or, in modern parlance, Alzheimer's disease— more than they fear cancer. And educated, informed people still fall prey to the pernicious prejudice of "ageism"—the bias against an individual simply because that person is old.

Ageism allows us to categorize the aged as somehow different from ourselves. This book sets out to show that, at least as far as brainpower is concerned, the aged are just like everyone else. Only 5 to 7 percent of persons over sixty-five years of age suffer from Alzheimer's disease or some other irreversible dementia; the remainder—the vast majority—are as capable as they ever were of learning, of interacting, of thinking and remembering. We still need to hear that message.

I have been living with the information you'll read in *The Myth of Senility* for the past five years. It has helped me better understand, and better value, the old people I have met along the way. I am thinking especially of the many guests at the seventy-fifth birthday party for Grandpa Ben (my husband's grandfather) who privately thanked me for the relief my optimistic message had brought them. No one had ever told these seventy- and eighty-year-olds the truth that they already knew—that advanced old age need not mean helplessness, dependence, fogginess, senility. And because no one had told them, they had each clung to their private knowledge tenuously, fearful that the next slipped thought, the next forgotten errand, could signal the beginning of an inevitable decline that only temporarily had eluded them.

The cold, clear afternoon of Grandpa Ben's party, tales poured from these old men and women—mostly women, since in this country women far outnumber men in this age group—about how they got through their active days, the notes and reminders and inventiveness they used to keep themselves busy. Anna, an old family friend, described a bedridden woman of ninety-four whom she had befriended as part of a Friendly Neighbors program at her synagogue. Anna was proud of this old woman and her sharp, crystalline mind—forgetting that, at the age of seventy-seven, she herself was defying the myth of senility.

That same afternoon my husband's other grandfather, Grandpa Maccy, also drove home the truth of how involved and intelligent the very old can be. Maccy had finally completed, he told me as the party ended, his book-length manuscript on the history of "miseducation" in America. The book was a culmination of Maccy's experience as a teacher, and his musings on the value of child-centered instruction in the schools. At the time he was working on it, he was nearly ninety.

Like many others interested in gerontology, I came to the field with a loving understanding of some wonderful older people. First were my grandparents, Joseph and Yetta Stern, whose physical ailments were no obstacle to their remaining alert, intelligent, and fiercely involved in our family's life until their deaths. Then were my grandparents by marriage, Max and Ida Henig and Ben and Jean Steinberg, who showed me, by glorious example, that older people can continue to read, write, think, and play a mean game of gin. Grandma Ida and Grandma Jean, both widowed now, continue to learn new skills of independence—like balancing their checkbooks—even in their eighties, and they still bake the best brownies and thumb cookies in the world.

I am grateful to these loved ones for being models for a healthy, alert old age. They were always in my mind as I researched, wrote, and updated this book. My love and thanks go to them, and to my parents, Sidney and Clare Marantz; my husband, Jeff; and our daughters, Jessica and Samantha. And thanks, too, to the people who helped bring the book to a new audience in its paperback edition, at a time when the public needs more than ever to know that "senility" is not inevitable: Marian Emr of the National Institute on Aging; and Lynn Seligman, my agent.

Acknowledgments

Acknowledgments are made to the following for their kind permission to reprint copyrighted material:

From "Generational and Cohort-specific Differences in Adult Cognitive Functioning: A 14-year Study of Independent Samples" by K. W. Schaie, G. V. Labouvie-Vief, B. U. Buech, in *Developmental Psychology*, Vol. 9, 1973, pp. 151–56, Figures 2 and 3. Copyright © 1973 by the American Psychological Association. Reprinted by permission.

Colin Blakemore, *Mechanics of the Mind.* Cambridge University Press, 1977.

Steel, Knight, and Feldman, Robert, "Diagnosing Dementia and its Treatable Causes." *Geriatrics*, March 1979.

Robert N. Butler, *Why Survive? Being Old in America.* Harper & Row, Publishers, Inc., 1975.

From *Collected Poems* by William Butler Yeats. Reprinted with permission of Macmillan Publishing Co., Inc. Copyright © 1928 by Macmillan Publishing Co., Inc., renewed 1956 by Georgie Yeats.

From B. Milner, S. Corkin, and H-L Teuber, "Further Analysis of the Hippocampal Amnesic Syndrome" in *Neuropsychologia*, Vol. 6. Reprinted with permission of Pergamon Press, Ltd.

From *Physiology and Cell Biology of Aging.* E. Cherkin, et al (editors). Copyright © 1979 by Raven Press.

From *Alzheimer's Disease*, R. Katzman, R. D. Terry, and K. L. Bick (editors). Copyright © 1978 by Raven Press.

From Jack Botwinick, *Aging and Behavior*, 2nd ed., p. 338. Copyright © 1978 by Springer Publishing Company, Inc., New York. Used by permission.

1

The Myth of Senility

Day after day Mama sat in the living room, ignored like an old armchair. If she asked for the television to be turned a little louder, her grandchildren would disregard her; if she asked them what they were learning in school, they would mumble something and run away. Mama's daughter-in-law had no time for her when Mama would invite her to sit for a while so they could do their knitting together; her son, who was always tired when he came home at night, would simply yawn when she suggested a game of cards. So Mama held her peace, grateful to her family for taking care of her now that her legs were giving out, and she learned to be ignored. Until one afternoon when she asked innocently, "What day is today?"

Suddenly, Mama was the center of attention. She had forgotten the day—what else was she forgetting? "Mama, don't you remember what you had for breakfast today?"

No, since her food had become so bland that there was really not much about breakfast worth remembering. "Mama, don't you remember what you did yesterday?" No, since the variation in routine had become so slight that her Tuesdays were usually very much like her Wednesdays. "Mama, don't you remember cousin Ethel's little girl?" No, since the children underfoot never stopped long enough for the old woman to meet them and talk to them.

Each blank look from Mama brought a new flurry of love and concern from her sons and daughters. It was the kind of attention she had not received in years, not since the days when she was strong enough to prepare a full-course dinner for eighteen people every Thanksgiving. And, without really meaning to, Mama began to learn to be forgetful. It was the only kind of behavior her family deemed important enough to pay attention to.

There was nothing wrong with Mama's mind. But her conversation gradually became so studded with "Where am I?" and "Who are you?" that she came to embody the stereotype of the confused, disoriented, forgetful old woman, the "senile" person expected to replace the mentally intact one after the age of seventy or seventy-five. The myth of senility—the expectation that old brains are invariably riddled with holes and cobwebs—had in Mama's case turned into what psychologists call a "self-fulfilling prophecy." Mama's family expected a certain kind of behavior—forgetfulness—from the old woman, so they reacted in a way that reinforced that behavior whenever it occurred, finally turning Mama into the very creature they had expected her to become.

The expectation of confusion and memory loss in the elderly leads people to treat the aged as though they cannot remember—and to interpret their own forgetful behavior, once they reach old age, as the first step toward that inevitable end. The myth of senility is the stuff of our nightmares. "I believe people fear senility, fear growing old and losing their minds and being put away, more than they fear cancer," says Robert Butler, chairman of the Ritter Department of Geriatrics and Adult Development at the Mount Sinai Medical Center in New York. A recent survey supports this: When asked how long they expected to live and how long they hoped to live, the vast majority of adults wished for shorter lifetimes than they thought awaited them. And in 1985 an Associated Press poll reported that less than half of those polled would like to live to be 100.

Despite our wishes, though, we are fast becoming a nation of old people. The seventy-five-plus age group—the so-called "old old," in whom the physical problems of age become common—is the fastest-growing today; it increased by 32 percent between 1970 and 1980, nearly four times the rate of growth for the population as a whole. The growth rate of the "oldest old"—Americans over eighty-five—is especially rapid, having grown by almost 60 percent between 1970 and 1980. By the year 2000, there may be as many as 35 million elderly Americans—an estimated 13 percent of the population—and roughly half of them are expected to be over seventy-five.

As the graying of America progresses, the political, economic, and medical institutions now serving the aged will have to adapt to make room for a population bulge at the end of life. The fight against ageism has been fought for years in the halls of Congress. The fight continues in the nation's medical schools, nursing homes, and doctors' offices, as a new breed of gerontologists takes arms against the myth of senility by trying to disentangle the effects of societal conditions and expectations from the physiological changes—both normal and abnormal—that occur in the aged brain.

This is also the task we have set for ourselves in this book. How much of senile behavior—loss of memory, loss of orientation, confusion, inability to calculate or reason—is the result of the aging process itself, and how much is the result of the situation into which we thrust the elderly? How much is caused by physiological changes in the brain and body, and how much by social influence? Such distinctions must remain uppermost in our minds as we set about the task of studying brain changes with age.

The widely held stereotype that all old people are forgetful, confused, "senile," damages not only the elderly but all of us. By categorizing persons over a certain age as mentally dull and incapable, society denies itself the brainpower of a generation—brainpower made all the more potent by a lifetime of experiences, perspective, and, in many fortunate cases, accumulated wisdom. On a resource-scarce planet, how can we squander the most precious resource of all: human intelligence?

The stereotype, of course, also does damage to the aged themselves. This happens in three ways. First, old people who show some of the normal mental changes of age, most prominently occasional forgetfulness, a slowing of thought, and a greater tendency to reminisce, become paralyzed with fear. As they observe the changes in their mental processes—which, although irksome, are usually harmless and can be adjusted for by subtle shifts in the environment—they become more and more convinced that this missed appointment, this forgotten telephone number, is the one that signals the beginning of the long slide toward senility and emptiness. And the myth of senility becomes a self-fulfilling prophecy—those who believe in it begin to act it out, and the myth once again appears to be true.

A second way in which the stereotype does damage is by denying to a large segment of the population the medical care they need to *avoid* becoming hopelessly senile. A significant number of elderly people—some say as many as 20 percent of the "old old"—experience dramatic changes in memory and state of alertness that are in fact medical emergencies. These people are not merely old, and their mental changes go beyond the mild changes that accompany healthy old age. They are sick, with underlying illnesses ranging from the commonplace—constipation, flu, anemia—to the exotic—occult hydrocephalus, hyperthyroidism or hypothyroidism, appendicitis. But if they and their families believe that senility is inevitable, they will disregard the importance of their only symptoms—forgetfulness and confusion—and will never see a physician. In these cases, the underlying, *and treatable*, illness remains undiagnosed, and the myth of senility can actually turn a reversible episode of senile behavior into a chronic, lifelong, disabling condition.

The senility stereotype also damages those individuals who *do* have a distinct neurological disease accurately labeled "senile dementia." Some 2 to 3 million middle-aged and elderly Americans are the victims of a disease called Alzheimer's disease—named after Alois Alzheimer, who first described it in 1906—and for them senility is not a myth but a cruel fact of life. The expectation of the profound hopelessness and mental emptiness attached to a diagnosis of Alzheimer's disease, however, does a great disservice to both victims and families. While the illness is progressive, incurable, and ultimately quite devastating, its progress can sometimes be stemmed, at least in the early stages, by a supportive environment. If everyone gives up on the patient with Alzheimer's disease, becoming overprotective and ever-watchful and denying him the independence and freedom needed to try and, if need be, fail, the patient's condition deteriorates rapidly. And oversolicitousness is the typical reaction of families of Alzheimer's disease patients when those families have always accepted the myth of senility.

Thus, societal and individual expectations can lead us to exacerbate normal mental changes, ignore abnormal ones, and overstate the dependency inherent in senile dementia when it does exist. Good students of the aging brain must, therefore, transcend the stereotype with which most Westerners were raised: that senility is inevitable; that anyone who lives long enough will eventually lose his memory, his wit, his mind. At the same time, they must learn not to be optimistic to the point of blindness to the mental and physical changes that *do* occur over time. Saying senility is not inevitable is not to say there is no such thing as senile dementia or the milder mental changes of old age. Being old is simply not the same as being young. But this does not mean that being old is something to be feared, avoided, or ignored.

Ageism and the Self-Sabotagers

A belief in the senility myth is the underside of the prejudice known as ageism. And ageism—a mixture of fear, revulsion, and stereotyping of the elderly—places its adherents in a quandary unique in the annals of bigotry. White racists do not suddenly wake up to find themselves black; male sexists cannot turn into women; but ageists are prejudiced against a minority group that they all one day will join. Thus, individuals who have grown up in our age-denying culture will grow old in an environment that fills them with self-loathing when they reach the magic age of sixty-five.

For some people, a way out of this predicament is the haven of the past, a retreat from the fact that the world and their place in it have changed now that they are old. For them, a descent into forgetfulness and "senility" is sparked, not by the unwitting reinforcement of friends and family or by the expectations of society, but by the old person himself, as if by choice. Robert Butler calls it "collaborating with their ostracizers." He says some people seem actually to choose to lose hold of their mental powers — just as some choose to let their bodies turn to fat — rather than fight to stay sharp and active. Either consciously or subconsciously, some old people will bend to the subtle social pressure to become crotchety, withdrawn, asexual, passive, dependent, depressed — not only because they believe they're supposed to, but because it is easier than fighting.

The difference between old people who yield to their psychic environments in this way, and those who remain feisty and independent despite all cues to do otherwise, may be a matter of basic personality. In the 1950s, Butler and others then working at the National Institute of Mental Health (NIMH) conducted a personality study that revealed differences between the self-sabotagers and the resisters, making it poignantly clear that society's most weak and vulnerable members are hardest hit by myths and stereotypes. The scientists administered Rorschach Inkblot Tests to their aged volunteers, and compared the results with those of American prisoners of war in Korea, some of whom had collaborated with the North Koreans. "It turned out that the volunteers who accepted all the stereotypes about age — that you're washed up, you're senile, you're not able to be physically active — reacted to those tests in the same way as those prisoners who had collaborated with the Communists," Butler says. "And those people who disagreed with what society expected from the aged followed the patterns shown by the prisoners who resisted collaboration." It may take an exceptional personality, then, to fight the social pressure to give in to the stereotype of senility. In a society that continually removes all sources of psychic strength from the elderly, stripping them of roles, income, and prestige, such a personality, even if it existed in the first place, is difficult to maintain into old age.

The progression from belief in the senility myth to the "self-sabotaging" Butler describes may be rooted as much in physiology as in psychology. When old people expect to become senile, each instance of forgetfulness makes them withdraw further into themselves. They become less likely to take part in conversations for fear of forgetting a word or a phrase; they become less willing to seek or keep a job out of certainty that they will fail somewhere. And as their intellectual world shrinks, as the challenges to which the brain is subjected become less demanding, the brain cells themselves may react, just as an unused muscle would, by shrinking, too.

Sensory deprivation has long been known to lead to the physical withering away of the brain, especially when it occurs during the early stages of development. Scientists are now discovering that sensory enrichment can have as profound an impact in the opposite direction—and that either environment, deprived or enriched, also can change the physical brain structure of the very old. Physiologist Marian Cleeves Diamond of the University of California at Berkeley, for example, spent fifteen years weighing the brains of aged rats reared in deprived environments and comparing them with the brains of their littermates raised in either standard or enriched environments. The rats in the enriched environments were found to have more brain cells, with more complex interconnections, than the rats who were deprived.

Most importantly, Diamond found that it's never too late for a brain to respond physically to changes in its environment: "Not only have chemical and anatomical studies demonstrated the plasticity of the cortex, but they have shown that the net weight of the cortex can increase or decrease at any age studied." Diamond says her findings are "encouraging and optimistic" regarding the fate of the human brain. If one's surroundings stay stimulating and supportive, her results imply, the environment can help bolster the size, complexity, and perhaps even the functioning of the brain in old age.

But when the aged are tossed from the mainstream of life—through either forced retirement, sudden impoverishment, or rejection on the basis of their physical deformities and disabilities—they disengage from the flow that had kept their minds alert and useful. The longer they sit, the more removed they become. "In terms of comparison with the functioning of an engine," says physician Claude Oster of the Rehabilitation Center of Southfield, Michigan, "it might be said that the brain is 'in neutral' when the patient is physically inactive, and becomes 'engaged' when the patient is in the standing position—the 'cephalopedal' reflex. The brain starts to function when the feet touch the floor." But people with nowhere to go are less likely even to stand up.

The Brain and Time

To begin our investigation of the mental changes that can accompany age, we first must view the brain as a physical organ that undergoes predictable physiological changes over time. In chapter 2, we will see just which structures the brain retains and which it loses—and we will try to draw some conclusions as to how these changes relate to the diminished capacity to respond quickly, especially to stress, that seems to characterize even the healthiest of the old.

Brain cells, or neurons, are among a handful of cells that do not replicate. By age two, we have all the neurons we will ever have—billions of them—and after the age of about thirty we begin steadily to lose them. At the same time that the brain becomes smaller, it also becomes lighter and wetter. The valleys between ridges of brain matter widen and deepen, and the brain is not quite the neat, efficient package it was in youth.

Losing neurons, though, need not mean losing function. In general, old age is a time of slower responsiveness and slower recall. But the vast majority of the elderly learn to compensate for that slowness. As memory totters, they write themselves notes: Have you locked the back door yet? Is the stove turned off? Take two yellow pills at 1:30. They use telephone books, calendars, diaries, lists more than they used to, and resort to tricks of expression—more simple sentences and fewer paragraphs, for example, might appear in their conversation and correspondence—when words begin to escape them. But they function, and function well.

Scientists can chart the actual decline that occurs in gray matter and white matter over the years—describing, as we shall in the next chapter, autopsy studies that include laborious cell counts, investigations of the complexity of the branching networks of cells, and measures of certain chemicals and chemical receptors—but they are hard-pressed to draw conclusions as to what that decline really means in terms of function. The brain, even the old brain, is such a resilient organ that many physical changes can escape unnoticed: The cells build a new pathway around dying cells, or grow new branches for sending and receiving messages. And beyond the resourcefulness of the neurons themselves is the always incalculable resourcefulness of the individual possessing the neurons. Perhaps Winston Churchill, whose brain is said to have been riddled with disease when he died at ninety-six, escaped mental debilitation through sheer pluck, through the strength of his mind, his constant intellectual activity, and his complex system of social, intellectual, and emotional support.

We shall see in the coming chapters that the old mind is like an old muscle: It must be used and challenged in order to function well. If housed within four empty walls and left to wither, the mind will indeed atrophy, roaming back into the past when it was put to good use and unable to snap back to the dreary present even when called upon to do so. But if enclosed in an environment that challenges, that stimulates, the mind not only will survive, it will grow. On the basis of studies such as Marian Cleeves Diamond's, neuroscientists conclude that the aged brain is capable of regenerating new branches, or dendrites, when the old dendrites wither away. These branches are necessary for communication from cell to cell; without them, the brain cannot do its work. Anatomists have noted a significant decline in the complexity of the interneuron connections— that is, in the number of dendrites per brain cell—as a person ages, an observation that implies a decreased ability to engage in mental excercises that demand intricate neural circuitry. But many of these interconnections seem capable of regrowth.

"Even though brain cells cannot divide and replicate," says Dr. Stanley Rapoport, chief of the Laboratory of Neurosciences at the National Institute on Aging (NIA), "many of the active undamaged cells in the elderly brain can grow more dendrites and axons, enhancing intercommunication. This phenomenon is called plasticity." Plasticity, he says, accounts for "maintenance of much normal intellectual functioning and brain metabolism with aging," despite the fact that many brain cells might have been lost over the years.

Plasticity may have a darker side. As Dr. Harold Brody, an anatomist at the State University of New York at Stony Brook, has noted, the new growth may occur haphazardly, and the neural circuitry can go haywire. "Regrowth of dendrites may introduce contacts with cells which are not within the original normal network, and may introduce aberrations in behavior not present earlier," he has said. But on balance, Brody told the Gerontological Society in 1979, it is far better to risk generating some crossed wires through a stimulating environment than to play it safe in a barren environment in which aged dendrites have no hope of replicating.

Robert Butler of the Mount Sinai Medical Center in New York takes a longer view of the relationship between external stimulation and the health of the brain. Unlike Brody, who explains improved mental functioning with a hypothesis about changes in the brain cells themselves, Butler, a psychiatrist by training, encompasses a whole psychosocial network in his explanation. "In work at the National Institute of Mental Health," he recounted in his Pulitzer Prize-winning book, *Why Survive?* "we observed the critical significance of the surrounding social environment upon mental health. The struggle for sheer survival needs, along with loneliness, idleness, and depression, absorb and bind considerable energy. Effective commitment to something outside oneself and the ability to act on one's own behalf are energizing."

Butler's orientation has its roots in the 1950s, when he participated in a unique study of healthy aged men sponsored by the National Institute of Mental Health (NIMH). The original investigation of forty-seven volunteers in 1957 and a follow-up of the survivors in 1968 form a work entitled *Human Aging* that shatters some long-held stereotypes about old age and its relationship to mental health and intellectual performance.

One of the most important findings of the NIMH Human Aging study is that general health status has a profound effect on mental capabilities. Although all forty-seven volunteers in 1957 were extraordinarily healthy for their age group (the average age was seventy-one), there was still a subgroup of twenty men who, after scrupulous, two-week-long medical examinations, were found to have minor physical abnormalities that produced no symptoms but could have proved troublesome later. This somewhat less healthy group—the men who seemed fine but had underlying problems of which they generally were unaware—differed mentally as well as physiologically from the twenty-seven "optimally healthy" men. Their brain function was found to have declined in comparison with the healthier group. The healthy group, in turn, gave a performance on intelligence tests and other measures of mental function that quite startled the investigators: they scored just about as high as the norm established for healthy young adults.

The Human Aging study laid the groundwork for the destruction of the myth of senility. The gradual scientific acceptance of its findings—that "senility" is not inevitable with age, but is associated with the physical debilitation that often accompanies age—was matched by a similar awakening occurring at about the same time among scientists studying cardiovascular disease. In the 1940s, most scientists had assumed that hardening of the arteries (atherosclerosis) was an inevitable part of growing old: if one lived long enough, one's blood vessels eventually became caked and clogged with fat. A small band of radicals put forth the idea that atherosclerosis was not an aging process but a disease process, one that could occur in persons of any age and that could someday be detected, prevented, and maybe even cured. Their views were roundly ridiculed—until the mid-1950s. Then, autopsy studies were first conducted on a group of soldiers killed in the Korean conflict. These studies turned up streaks of fatty deposits in the arteries of men as young as twenty-two. Clearly, the process of atherosclerosis had started long before the other physical concomitants of "normal aging." Today, we generally view atherosclerosis as a disease, not a consequence of age, and we accept the fact that diet, exercise, family history, and certain drugs can determine whether we develop atherosclerosis or escape it even in very old age.

A comparable evolution of knowledge has taken place in the last twenty-five years about senility. During that span, intelligence and memory tests have been redesigned and reinterpreted to confirm what the Human Aging study found in 1957: that, in general, healthy old people lose neither their minds nor their memories. As we shall see in chapter 3, gerontologists today are issuing optimistic reports about the life of the mind in its last years. Among their findings are that

- most old people remain throughout life as intelligent as they ever were;
- when intelligence test scores do decline with age, speed of performance is usually an important factor;
- on self-paced tests, even those involving the incor-

poration of new types of abstract information, old people perform better than they do on timed tests, and they usually perform almost as well as young people do;

- on certain tests of accumulated knowledge, such as vocabulary tests, people actually perform better as they get older;
- scores on intelligence tests decline less over time for people with a higher educational level and higher initial scores than for less educated or less intelligent peers, either because the education itself provides some protective effect, or because it is associated with a lifestyle in which the mind is better used;
- many people seem to become more forgetful with age, but this may be due primarily to a slowdown in the retrieval of information, rather than to a total obliteration of the memory trace.
- if old persons are taught to store new information more efficiently, their ability to retrieve it later improves significantly.

These findings have brought us a long way from the days when everyone, professionals and laypersons alike, believed that chronic, irreversible brain disease — usually called "hardening of the arteries of the brain" — was inevitable with age. Today, most experts in gerontology realize that senile dementia is a distinct disease affecting a small percentage of the aged population, and they think that it might one day be preventable or even curable. Moreover, they are beginning to recognize senile symptoms as occasionally being not the result of a brain disease at all, but the manifestation of illnesses affecting other parts of the body.

Pseudosenility

The ravages of time, even when they do not seriously interfere with an old person's ability to live in a relatively
stable, familiar, and supportive environment, can wreak
havoc with that same person's ability to cope with stress.
The stress may be socially induced—loss of a loved one,
sudden hospitalization, forced relocation—or it may be
physically induced—a heart attack, an infection, a long
bout of diarrhea or constipation. Because old people are
often juggling a variety of compensatory mechanisms in
order to maintain mental functioning in the face of the ordinary physiological losses of age, the final stress—which
looks harmless enough to an outsider, and would indeed be
harmless to a younger, more intact individual—may be
enough to topple the delicate balance. Thus the old person,
as the psychiatrists say, "decompensates," entering into a
murky netherworld which we shall explore in chapter 4:
the world of pseudosenility.

A long list of physical illnesses, among them those that
produce some of the most striking and easy-to-spot symptoms in the young, leads to few common symptoms in the
elderly. Heart attacks are one dramatic example. "In acute
myocardial infarction, less than 40 percent of older patients present with the classic findings of heart attack:
chest pain and shortness of breath," says Thomas Kalchthaler, medical director of the St. Joseph's Nursing Home
in Yonkers, New York. "Many will present with either confusional states, or weakness and dizziness." Many other
conditions also produce only vague complaints, usually including confusion, in the aged: low blood sugar, hyperthyroidism, appendicitis, severe infections, dehydration, malnutrition, vitamin deficiency, anemia, kidney failure.

As long as the general population believes that confusion is acceptable—indeed, inevitable—in the elderly, thousands of old persons with such straightforward medical problems as endocrine deficiencies or chronic anemia will never even be brought to a physician's office. As long as physicians, too, continue to accept the myth of senility, they will be quick to pigeonhole those confused elderly patients they do see as irreversibly senile, and will miss the 20 percent or so suffering merely from pseudosenility—a condition in which underlying treatable disorders create symptoms that look like senile dementia. This cavalier diagnosis changes the old man or old woman from a sick, potentially curable patient, into a victim, trapped in a vicious circle of dependence and disorientation that ultimately turns him or her into just the creature the senility myth predicted. The mind, unnourished and unused, turns sour, and the illness, which began as a reversible disease elsewhere in the body, eventually becomes a full-blown chronic brain disease. The old man or old woman, by now perhaps forced to live in a mental institution or nursing home, becomes another statistic—a statistic that seems to confirm the "inevitability" of senilty. But to the extent that this senility is inevitable, it is so only because the gerontophobia of Western culture has turned it into a self-fulfilling prophecy.

Who Goes Senile?

Nothing in the anatomical stars decrees that by a certain age we will all lose our minds. With the right kind of social and emotional support—and some common sense, native intelligence, and good luck thrown in—most of us can live mentally fulfilling lives until we die. We may forget more than we once did, and may have more trouble learning new languages or new abstract concepts, but with patience on the part of both the teacher and the taught, almost anything is possible—at any age. After all, the Roman statesman Cato is said to have taught himself Greek at the age of eighty. The figures confirm this optimistic outlook: Of the 27 million Americans now over the age of sixty-five, only about 7 percent show serious intellectual impairment, and only 10 percent exhibit mild to moderate loss of memory.

The odds, then, favor a healthy, functioning old age for most Americans. Even for those who become so confused and disoriented that they need a doctor's care, the odds are perhaps as high as 1 in 5 that the confusion can be cleared through vigorous treatment of an underlying medical problem.

But there will always be a small portion of the elderly population who play the odds and lose. For many Americans—current estimates run as high as 2 to 3 million—senile symptoms are real and irreversible. According to Dr. John Blass of the Burke Rehabilitation Center in White Plains, New York, approximately 10 percent of dementia in persons over sixty-five can be ascribed to brain tumor, Parkinson's disease, psychiatric illness, or one of a handful of rare neurological diseases such as Huntington's disease, Pick's disease, Creutzfeld-Jakob disease, and Korsakoff's psychosis. Another 17 percent can be traced to what is known as "multi-infarct dementia," the illness once mistakenly called "hardening of the arteries of the brain" that is an outgrowth of vascular problems (hypertension, aneurysms, heart disease, or arteriosclerosis) elsewhere in the body. In 7 percent of demented older patients, Blass estimates, the cause is unclear. And in approximately 66 percent of demented older patients, he says, the cause is Alzheimer's disease, either alone or in combination with multi-infarct dementia.

Because Alzheimer's disease strikes some 2 million Americans, with an age-related incidence that rises to 20 percent of all those who live past the age of eighty, it is especially important as part of the overall picture of the aged brain. It is an awesome disease, one that progresses inexorably toward loss of memory, so that in its late stages the victim may forget names of close friends and relatives, or even his or her own name. It also progresses toward disorientation, inability to think, to reason, to calculate, and, finally, to perform the simple chores of everyday life. At its most severe, the disease progresses rapidly, leading to death within five years; more commonly, improved medical care for Alzheimer's patients means they may live with their disease for a decade or more. Persons with Alzheimer's disease usually are institutionalized in their final years, and they die not so much of the brain illness itself as of the side effects of the immobility to which they are relegated—pneumonia, for example, or malnutrition. Robert Katzman, chairman of the Department of Neurosciences at the University of California in San Diego, and chairman of the medical advisory board of the Alzheimer's and Related Disorders Association, has estimated that Alzheimer's disease accounts for 100,000 to 120,000 deaths a year, ranking it as the fourth or fifth most deadly disease in the nation.

Alzheimer's disease is characterized by two typical changes in the brain: pairs of neuron fibers twisted around each other, called neurofibrillary tangles; and clusters of the tangles and other abnormal tissues, called neuritic plaques. The tangles and plaques seem directly to cause the mental infirmities of Alzheimer's disease: they occur in greatest number in the hippocampus and the cerebral cortex, two regions of the brain associated with memory and intellectual functioning. But not everyone with plaques and tangles becomes senile—and not everyone labeled senile has plaques and tangles. The brains of scores of alert, active old men and women have been found to be chock-full of brain lesions at autopsy, while the brains of some individuals who die in nursing homes, diagnosed as "demented" and showing no spark of intelligence or memory, are relatively free of the debris of Alzheimer's disease at autopsy.

Is Alzheimer's disease hereditary? The scientists still are not sure. The uncertainty of the verdict is especially worrisome since the symptoms of Alzheimer's rarely appear before the age of fifty, and often not until the sixties or seventies—long past the years of deciding about childbearing. If Alzheimer's disease is indeed carried on the genes, how can a rational trade-off be made between granting life, with a possible legacy of demise some fifty or sixty years hence, and denying life altogether? In chapter 6, we shall meet one family from suburban Philadelphia who is grappling with just such a decision.

According to Dr. Marshal Folstein of Johns Hopkins University, there probably is a gene for Alzheimer's disease —and it is probably a dominant gene. Ordinarily, gene dominance means that everyone having the gene expresses it. This is what occurs with the genes for eye color: a person with one brown-eyed and one blue-eyed gene always has brown eyes, because brown is dominant and blue is recessive. But because the Alzheimer's gene is expressed only late in life, and probably needs certain environmental triggers to be expressed, only about half of the people carrying the gene are likely to develop the disease. Folstein estimates that a person with the Alzheimer's disease gene has a 5 to 1 chance of dying of some other cause before the gene is expressed.

At the present time, Alzheimer's disease is incurable. The progression of brain degeneration cannot be stopped;

even the symptoms of forgetfulness and disorientation cannot be eased. As we shall see in chapter 7, some physicians have prescribed certain drugs, such as Hydergine, papaverine, and magnesium pemoline, to counter the memory loss and personality change that are part of Alzheimer's disease; the results so far have been mixed. Others recommend dietary supplements, such as lecithin, choline, and nicotinic acid; again, results are mixed. Until the cause of the disease is found, attempts at treatment will probably remain only patch-up jobs, and patients and their families will view the diagnosis of Alzheimer's disease as a sentence of eventual mental emptiness.

The rapidity with which the mind goes blank, though, may still be modifiable, as socially oriented researchers into Alzheimer's disease are beginning to learn. Supportive family surroundings, a place to go each day, a task to do, can help persons with Alzheimer's disease remain functional for far longer than they would have had they been tucked away early into a nursing home. Formal techniques such as "reality orientation," tried successfully in nursing homes around the country, and less structured attempts at support such as day care centers, continued employment of some sort, or frequent social interaction, may defer the day when the person with Alzheimer's disease feels useless and helpless. If nothing else, such activities seem to help dispel one of the most troublesome concomitants of Alzheimer's disease: depression.

Old Age in the Future

Depression, Alzheimer's disease, and pseudosenility present similar problems to the aged, who have trouble distinguishing among possible causes of certain mental changes

21

over time. Doctors also have trouble in the "differential diagnosis" of elderly patients who look merely "senile." Physicians in the past were not taught about the particular medical needs of old people; their medical school professors tended to disregard the aged as a generally unresponsive, uninteresting, unrewarding group of patients, so the many possible causes of senile behavior usually were not included in the curriculum. But geriatric medicine has suddenly become a popular field of study. Many medical students and younger professors now recognize that geriatrics provides a chance to bring to bear a host of interdisciplinary skills in their dealings with patients. They are aware that treatment of the aged demands the most of their clinical competence, and forces them to enlist the help of nurses, social workers, physical therapists, psychologists, and community activists. They are aware, too, that the bulk of their patients in the future are going to be old. As we shall see in chapter 8, estimates are that a doctor entering almost any field of medical practice today can expect from 40 to 60 percent of his patients to be over age sixty-five, and this proportion is likely to increase in years ahead.

Medicine's long-standing disregard of the aged has done them a great disservice, and is in part responsible for the widespread belief that "senility" is inevitable with age. Doctors have for years perpetuated this myth rather than take the additional time and expense to investigate just what might be causing an old man's confusion or an old woman's sudden disorientation. "What do you expect at your age?" has been the refrain heard in doctors' offices and hospitals across the country. But with the slow but steady growth of geriatric training in medical school — as of 1982, about two-thirds of all medical schools taught geriatrics in one form or another, and all are expected to join the ranks by 1995—this picture is likely to change. Not only information but also an attitude must be transmitted to impressionable medical students that will make them eager to accept the challenge of caring for the aged. Part of this new attitude will require a redefinition of medical success.

In chapter 9, we shall investigate an alternate route for arriving at medical success—not through the medical model, but through changes in the individual's living environment. Some gerontologists are studying simple tricks and devices for making old persons' homes safe places in which to be forgetful, thus minimizing the hazards resulting from memory loss and making it less likely that the milder mental changes of age will require institutionalization in the long run. Indeed, environmental manipulation has met with some success in more severe brain problems of age as well, such as Alzheimer's disease. Although a brightly colored room or a more sensible arrangement of furniture does not halt the inevitable progression of Alzheimer's, and seems not even to slow the loss of intellectual functioning, such changes in the surroundings can improve a patient's emotional outlook and sociability, which are no small matters in influencing quality of life.

These more innovative approaches to care of the elderly are being undertaken in part because traditional methods have proved insufficient, and in part because the needs of the future are likely to be greater than any we have known. The number of persons with Alzheimer's disease and also of those suffering from the normal slowing and forgetfulness of very old age increases as the number of the aged increases. And in response to the crush of demographics, politicians and researchers have responded with new approaches to research into the mental changes of age.

Chapter 10 will outline some of these new approaches, most of them centered at the National Institute on Aging

(NIA). NIA sponsors a broad range of projects in the dementias—including population studies, behavioral research, and studies at the cellular level—that reflect the emerging importance of senile dementia on the nation's research agenda. At a time when Congress is cutting back on money appropriated for the nation's biomedical research enterprise, NIA is one of the few agencies that have been receiving more money to award to scientists interested in studying essential questions in aging. Among those questions, some of the most frequently asked are the very questions we ask ourselves in this book: How much of senile behavior is the result of the aging process itself and how much the result of the situation into which we thrust the elderly? How much is caused by physiological changes in the brain and body and how much by social influences? And, perhaps most important, how much of the normal mental changes of age, and of the pathological changes that are the result of disease, can be treated, reversed, and one day even prevented?

᛫ *2* ᛫

Brain Changes with Age: Form vs. Function

Old brains, like old faces and old bodies, look different from young ones. The brain becomes smaller, lighter, wetter than it was in youth—a gradual, progressive change that probably begins in adolescence. There are fewer brain cells, or neurons, in the aged brain, although the loss of cells occurs at different rates in different sections. Some areas of the brain remain intact throughout a lifetime; other areas have lost as many of one-half their original number of neurons by the age of ninety or so. In the same way one's body loses tone with advanced age, so too does one's brain. The valleys, or gyri, that separate the ridges of brain matter become wider and deeper, and the entire brain pulls in from its encasement, the cortical mantle, like a sagging skin.

Losing neurons, though, need not mean losing function. And the exact nature of the relation between form and

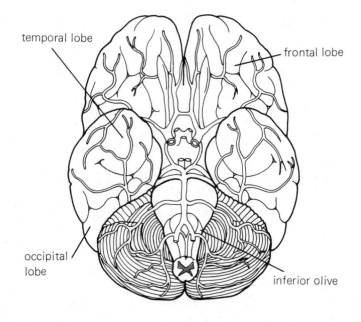

temporal lobe

frontal lobe

occipital lobe

inferior olive

1. The physical structure of the brain.

function still eludes the grasp of researchers in neurology and pathology. Realizing that the physical structure of the brain (see illustration) plays an important role in determining behavior, students of the mind realize, too, that the brain is not absolute in its control. True, physical changes in the brain have been shown directly to cause changed behavior, intelligence, sleep patterns, and memory. But people with severely damaged brains are sometimes able to live long and normal lives, while others who have acted strangely for years turn out to have brains that, to a pathologist, look normal.

This paradox is compounded in the aging brain, since no one knows yet which changes are inevitable with age and which are the result of diseases that often accompany aging. Like investigators of aging elsewhere in the body, investigators of the aging brain still haven't agreed on whether the distinction between normal aging and disease is one of degree or of kind.

"One of the greatest strides that neuroscientists have made in the last few decades," says Carl Eisdorfer, professor of psychiatry and neuroscience at Albert Einstein School of Medicine in New York, "is a change in their conception of the brain as an electrical system to the brain as a plumbing system." The traditional analogy of the electrical impulses of the brain leaping from one neuron to another is not entirely correct. With the consistency of Jell-O, the human brain is far more liquid than this image would suggest. The transmittal of messages in the brain is performed mostly, not by little sparks, but by the secretion of neurotransmitters, specialized chemicals with which impulses may hitch a ride across the gap separating one brain cell from another.

Just about all the changes that have been demonstrated in the aged brain are thought to interfere with this transmittal process somewhere along the line. There are fewer neurons, and each neuron is less efficient than it once was; there is a decrease in the nutritious extracellular space between neurons, which ordinarily eggs on the impulse from one cell to another; the number of regenerating structures within the remaining neurons sharply declines; there is a marked decrease in some of the most important neurotransmitters, the ferrymen of the system; and there is a proliferation of lesions and foreign substances—plaques, tangles, non-neuronal brain cells, pieces of pigment—that tend to plug up the works in one way or another.

It is hard to draw many conclusions about cognitive function from the physical changes that have been observed in the aged brain. The brain is a remarkably resilient organ, and it can withstand enormous physical trauma without seriously impairing behavior. In the 1930s, for example, large portions of the cerebral cortex, long considered the seat of higher intelligence, were removed in persons with severe epilepsy—yet these "decorticated" patients maintained much of the intellectual capacity thought to be housed in the brain sections that had been removed!

In many ways, it would be a liberating finding, for young and old alike, if physical brain changes could be specifically linked to cognitive changes—a goal of many of today's neurologists. If nothing else, such a connection would remove some of the guilt now felt by the aged and their families when old folks don't function as well as they used to. And if scientists can pinpoint which anatomical changes create which aberrant behavior, perhaps someday they can take steps to prevent those changes in the first place, or to correct them when the aberrant behavior shows up.

So we must recognize, as we review the findings of physical changes in the brain with age, that older brains are indeed different. While the resiliency of the mind should keep us from becoming fatalistic about these changes, and while the tenuousness of the form-function relationship should make us wary of drawing too literal a conclusion about aged behavior, we must also avoid overoptimism. Certain common changes in aged behavior—primarily a slowing in the processing of information through the central nervous system, and therefore a slowing of just about every function the old person engages in—can indeed be explained by changes in the aged brain. The trick now is to discover which brain changes account for which behavioral changes.

Neuron Countdown

Harold Brody of the State University of New York at Buffalo was the first scientist systematically to count the number of cells at different ages in certain areas of the brain. The task was as awesome as counting stars in the night sky, since the number of neurons in the average brain is thought to be about the same as the number of stars in the Milky Way—more than 15 billion. Brody counted the cells appearing in brain slices from various regions of the brain that were taken from people ranging in age from newborn to ninety years old. His only aid in the effort was a counting grid mounted to the eyepiece of his microscope.

The lengthy efforts paid off, because Brody found some surprising news. Although there was indeed a marked decrease in the number of neurons in the aged brains as opposed to the young ones, the decrease was not consistent from one part of the brain to another. And, perhaps more important, the cell loss was not an isolated function of old age; in fact, the greatest rate of neuronal death in the cerebral cortex—the seat of "higher" intellectual functioning—occurred between birth and about the age of thirty. After that, neuronal loss continued, but at a slower pace than before.

Some parts of the brain don't seem to lose neurons at all. The number of cells in the vestibular nucleus, a small group of neurons in the brainstem that helps maintain head posture, does not diminish with age. Neither does the number of cells in the inferior olive, a larger group of cells in the hindbrain that is associated with the motor control of the cerebellum. Other parts of the brain lose a considerable number of neurons. The cortex is the most dramatic example; another is the locus ceruleus, a group of pigmented nerve cells known to affect sleep stages and perhaps intelligence. And scientists have found a cell loss of nearly 30 percent after age fifty in the region of the brain called the hippocampus.

The fate of the hippocampus is perhaps the most important structural change in the aged brain. It is in regard to this region, tucked inside the folds of the cortex, that scientists feel most comfortable about making connections between brain structure and behavior, since the hippocampus has been widely studied and is generally considered to be the seat of learning, memory, and perhaps even pleasure. Dozens of studies on animals, and on one ill-fated man we will meet in the next chapter, have shown that total loss of these brain cells can result in total loss of conscious memory.

Even in as carefully studied a region as the hippocampus, though, neuroscientists still are not sure just which cognitive changes can be expected to result from hippocampal damage. In fact, they have been forced to retreat to a prior question—a question they had thought was long settled—and find out just how much hippocampal damage occurs in the aged brain. Since the 1960s, when the husband-wife team of Madge Scheibel and Arnold Scheibel first counted hippocampal cells in their lab at the University of California at Los Angeles, the conventional wisdom had been that as many as 20 to 40 percent of the cells were lost by the time an individual reached the age of ninety. More important, the Scheibels found that the cells by that age had lost up to 80 percent of their dendrites—tiny, hairlike filaments needed to detect and transmit nerve impulses through the neuron, and needed to carry nutrients to the brain cell as well (see illustration). The denudation of this "dendritic arbor," likened to a tree's loss of leaves, then twigs, then branches and limbs, was considered by the Scheibels, and other anatomists, to be a precursor to the death of brain cells.

But Paul Coleman, a neuroanatomist at the University of Rochester, has questioned these findings. "Growth is not the exclusive province of early development," he says. "Regressing neurons notwithstanding, the net effect of advancing age, at least early in old age, is dendritic growth." Coleman says that new computer-assisted methods of cell counting at dendrite visualization reveal a pattern of increased arborization in certain regions of the brain. In the aging brain, he concludes, both growth and decline occur concurrently. He further concludes that during early old age, the brain cells that are growing dendrites are more plentiful; during late old age, the dying cells predominate. It is only late in life that the balance tips away from growth and toward overall decline.

Even if cell loss were to be agreed upon down to the hundredth place, however, we still would not know precisely how these brain changes translate into behavioral

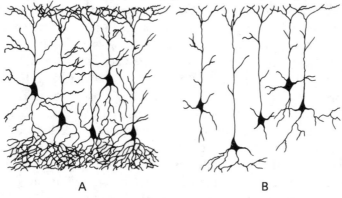

           A   B

2. *The loss of dendritic branching with age. Figure A is from a young neuron, figure B is from a senile brain.*

changes. Loss of neurons—even the most important neurons, whose roles in intelligence have been carefully described—does not necessarily lead to problems. As we have seen, epileptic patients in the 1930s whose cortexes were removed functioned quite well without this section of the brain, which is considered the seat of higher intelligence. Conversely, old people with the most severely debilitating changes in cognitive function—those suffering from Alzheimer's disease—have the same number of neurons as do nondiseased old people who function quite normally. Contrary to previous teaching, which said the mental deficits of Alzheimer's disease were caused by a rapid loss of brain cells, brains of Alzheimer's disease victims have been shown to have the same number of neurons as do the brains of normal, age-matched controls.

Clearly, the relationship between cell loss and mental decline is neither simple nor direct. It must be inferred, usually through a series of hypotheses and logical deductions, which leads scientists to believe that the large loss of brain cells in particular regions of the aged brain may contribute to some cognitive decline. In regard to one such region, the locus ceruleus, the reasoning goes like this: The locus ceruleus is thought to be responsible for maintaining sleep patterns in the healthy adult. An estimated 20 to 30 percent of the neurons in this region are lost in the normal aged brain. This cell loss may explain, at least in part, the changes in sleep patterns that have been observed in elderly people. Not only do the aged generally sleep fewer hours per day—often spreading these hours over several catnaps rather than in one nighttime stretch—but the quality of the sleep decreases, too. In a typical night's sleep, an old person experiences more light sleep and less Stage 4 (deep) and REM (actively dreaming) sleep. This tendency is further aggravated when old people are placed on sedatives, drugs that are, ironically, often prescribed for persons complaining of sleeplessness. The loss of deep sleep is important, since excessive deprivation of Stage 4 sleep—in healthy research subjects who were awakened whenever they trailed off into deep sleep—has been shown to be associated with cognitive dysfunction. Thus the tentative conclusion is: a loss of brain cells in the locus ceruleus may account for some cognitive dysfunction in the elderly.

Why do some neurons die off with age? Some scientists theorize that the rejuvenating mechanism that keeps each cell functioning somehow breaks down as time goes by. Unlike all other body cells, neurons don't divide; but like all cells, even neurons regenerate. As Nobel laureate Christian de Duve has put it, old brains are like old cities. "Whereas the town as a whole may go back many centuries, most of its buildings have been destroyed and reconstructed many times." Similarly, the content of neurons may be only a few days or weeks old, even though the neuron itself is as old as the individual.

But like the fate of old cities, the fate of old brains depends on their ability to maintain an inflow of new components. Just as city services and neighborhood vitality can help explain why one section of town becomes run-down while another becomes chic, the workings of the brain's own rejuvenator—a cell part called a lysosome—can determine whether a neuron lives or dies. In many old neurons, it seems, these lysosomes—the sanitation workers of the system—have become old and sluggish, and they rarely come by anymore to pick up the trash. This leads to the accumulation of so much waste material, called lipofuscin, that nothing can get by, and the commerce of doing the brain's work is permanently stalled.

33

Lipofuscin—Age Spots on the Brain

It's yellow, insoluble, coarsely granular. The lipids within it are abnormal, with ends of molecules attached to middles of other molecules in a rigid, contorted fashion. Some have described the material as a junkyard, where undegradable waste from broken-down cell membranes and other cell components accumulate. The picture of this compound, lipofuscin, isn't a pretty one.

Lipofuscin is the pigment that accounts for the brown "liver spots" on the hands and faces of older people. And it is found increasingly in the cell body of most neurons as they age. Although scientists are uncertain just how damaging to the neuron this age pigment can be, a few observations are significant. Those brain cells with the greatest amount of lipofuscin have been shown to have correspondingly fewer components needed to synthesize protein in the brain. In addition, scientists have found that the more lipofuscin a brain cell has, the less RNA it has—and the genetic compound RNA has been shown to play a major role in the formation and storage of memory.

Clearly, then, the pigment inhibits at least some of the work of the neuron. Christian de Duve theorizes that its accumulation is accounted for largely by the breakdown in the functioning of the lysosome, the cell component responsible for digestion of all regenerating cell parts. Lysosomes, the sanitation workers of the brain, begin to lose their capacity for autophagy (or self-destruction) as they age, and so the by-product of this waste metabolism begins to accumulate in places where it should not. Old lysosomes have lost an essential enzyme needed for autophagy, which renders the by-product indigestible. Having nowhere to go, it remains in the lysosome in the form of the pigment lipofuscin. The pigment builds up, and the lysosome swells to contain more and more of it. Within the confines of the neuronal space, the lysosome's growth means something else must give way. Scientists think that the neuron's protein-making apparatus, called the endoplasmic reticulum, is the first to go.

"In view of the role played by lysosomes in the turnover process," de Duve observes, "it may be said that the aging of lysosomes is the price cells have to pay for rejuvenating their constituents." The price could be great. Lysosomal storage diseases such as Tay-Sachs, Niemann-Pick, and Hurler's disease involve the pile-up of indigestible materials in the lysosome—materials that are indigestible not because of age but because an essential enzyme has been missing since birth. Victims of these storage diseases generally die within a few years. "It seems reasonably sure from these experiments of nature, fortunately of rare occurrence, that overloading of the lysosomes is sufficient in itself to bring about severe cellular damage, to the point of causing lethal impairments of function," says de Duve. "This is particularly true in neurons, where lack of expansion space causes any increase in lysosome volume necessarily to take place at the expense of other cell constituents."

As with most other neurological observations, the relationship between the buildup of lipofuscin in the brain and the death of brain cells is paradoxical. Although it is tempting to conclude that as the age pigment accumulates in the lysosome, the cell is kept from doing its work and therefore dies, the cause-and-effect relationship is in fact unclear. For one thing, scientists cannot even agree on whether the pigment is, in the end, good for you or bad for you. "This confusion may be partly due to the lack of direct evidence on the functions of the cell with and without the pigment," says Kalidas Nandy of Boston University, an ex-

pert in lipofuscin. The state of knowledge is still so ele-
mentary that researchers are not yet sure whether lipofuscin itself is a cause of learning and memory problems in
some old people or whether, as Nandy suggests, it "represents the ashes after the fire" of a lifetime of wear and tear.

Similarly, some scientists are beginning to think that
the age pigment doesn't kill cells at all, but rather is the
badge worn by cells able to win their battle for survival.
This idea was prompted by the confusing finding that the
hardiest parts of the brain seem to be the regions with the
greatest concentrations of lipofuscin. In the group of neurons known as the inferior olive, for example, lipofuscin
begins to accumulate in early childhood; by old age, the inferior olive has a higher concentration of lipofuscin than
any other brain region. And yet, the olive is one of the
regions of the brain in which neurons virtually never die.

Pathologist Robert Terry of the University of California
at San Diego has a hypothesis for this apparent anomaly:
Perhaps some neurons are simply more susceptible than
others to the lethal effects of lipofuscin. Or, he suggests, it
may not be the lipofuscin at all that is lethal, but one of its
metabolic precursors. Those cells that die, according to
this theory, are the ones that cannot convert the dangerous
precursor into the relatively harmless form of lipofuscin.
Those cells that survive are the ones that can—which would
explain why lipofuscin exists in large amounts in the hardiest survivors.

When Brains Bounce Back

Some of the changes observed in older brains may not be
the result of death and decline at all, but the outcome of
the brain's ability to compensate for its losses. Sometimes,

the efforts at compensation seem to work to the old person's advantage. Sometimes, the compensation is slightly awry, and the result is, sadly, simply a further clogging up of the brain's transporation system.

One example of successful compensation is the change that has been observed in the blood vessels of the aged brain. Scientists at the Sandoz Institute of Basic Medical Research in Basel, Switzerland, found that these tiny vessels change in size and shape with age: they become wider, longer, and closer together in relation to the size of the brain itself. The Swiss researchers hypothesize that the changes might be necessary for continued good functioning. Since blood flow in the brain seems generally to decline with age, they say, the proliferation of the brain's blood vessels may "completely compensate" for this reduced blood flow, allocating a sufficient amount of blood to reach the brain's cells—already decreased in number because of the normal cell loss that accompanies age.

Other compensatory reactions, though, seem to work less well in the aged. When a young person's brain is "insulted," or attacked, through infection, trauma, or some other external force, a type of brain cell called the glial cell is known to rally to the brain's defense. Glial cell proliferation, or gliosis, is a frequent part of brain infection in the young, and the assemblage of these tiny cells—one-seventh the size of a neuron—is thought to provide the nutrients and blood supply needed to ward off the attack.

Perhaps as a reaction to the generalized brain "insults" of age, gliosis also occurs almost without exception in the aged brain. These cells, which ordinarily act as a nest for neurons to keep each one supplied with blood and protein, are believed to contribute to brain impulse conduction and to the viability of the individual neuron. But the gliosis of old age is thought not to enhance this protective function,

37

but simply further to plug up the works in an already compromised brain.

The glial cells involved in the growth spurt of old age are probably abnormal cells—which accounts for the apparent failure of the compensatory effort. The Swedish scientist Holger Hyden studied the genetic composition of the glial cells found prominently in the brains of persons with Parkinson's disease, a neurological disorder that in many ways resembles other brain diseases of old age. Many of the brain changes in Parkinson's disease, which usually strikes people over sixty, are also found in normal old brains; gliosis is one of those changes. Early in the disease process, Hyden found, the RNA that carried the glial cell's basic genetic code was "highly aberrant"; it was not until the disease progressed that the RNA of the neuron was also found to be deranged. "To judge from the time sequence," notes psychiatrist Antonia Vernadakis in a summary of Hyden's findings, "the biochemical error first develops in the glia, which then seem to influence neurons both biochemically and functionally."

Another compensatory trick that may backfire is a lower threshold of arousal in the aged brain. To adjust for the fact that impulses are harder to detect with fewer neurons, reduced dendritic branches, and (as we shall see in the next section) a lesser amount of neurotransmitters, the aged brain may somehow see to it that its level of reactivity is turned up a notch, rather like increasing the volume on a television dial. But this increased volume, which tunes in to unimportant impulses as well as important ones, could result in what some scientists have called "neural noise." In a "noisy" brain, it becomes harder to discriminate new impulses from the generalized background hum. Thus, this misguided compensation could account for some confusion and slowing down in the elderly thought process.

Neurotransmitters: The Ferrymen Disappear

Another explanation for the slowing seen with normal aging is the decrease in the levels of several important neurotransmitters in the older brain. In the last fifteen years, scientists have discovered some thirty chemicals that may serve as "ferrymen" in the brain's transport system, moving signals from one cell to another across the moats known as synapses. Each neuron seems designed to manufacture or receive only one neurotransmitter; thus, the level of a particular transmitter in the aged brain reflects the presence or absence of a particular kind of neuron and is a key to piecing together the story of the brain's structural fate.

A neurotransmitter system comprises a precursor enzyme, which manufactures the chemical; the neurotransmitter itself; and an inhibiting compound that is released when the transmitter level gets too high. In the aged brain, at least three of these systems seem to go awry. The most significant system to fail is the cholinergic system.

The cholinergic system, which makes the transmitter acetylcholine, seems crucial in the formation and storage of memory. Proof of this lies in experiments such as those performed by David Drachman at Northwestern University, in which drugs interfering with the cholinergic system produced, in healthy college students, memory impairments that mimicked the changes seen in old age. Since Drachman's early studies in the mid-1970s, scientists have found an explanation for the phenomenon he observed: Most old people, like the students in the experiment, suffer a loss of brain chemicals involved in the cholinergic system.

The precursor enzyme in this system, choline acetyltransferase, has been shown to decline by as much as 70 percent in the typical aged brain. This means that the transmitter itself, acetylcholine, probably undergoes a parallel decline. Peter Davies of Albert Einstein College of Medicine in New York believes that this decrement is a result of disease, not of normal aging, since "a few fortunate individuals in their nineties retain their choline acetyltransferase activity to the bitter end—and they also maintain their intellectual function until the day they die." Still, a significant decline in this enzyme is the rule in the aged population, so if it is due to illness, it is probably an illness that strikes almost all older people.

Cholinergic system disruption has been implicated in at least one illness affecting the aged: Alzheimer's disease, the subject of chapters 5 and 6, which is the most common form of "senile dementia." In patients with Alzheimer's disease, the level of choline acetyltransferase plummets to just 10 percent of its earlier level. "In these patients," says Davies, "a clear correlation has been observed between the loss of choline acetyltransferase and the degree of psychometric impairment."

Other important neurotransmitters have also been shown to decline with age. Transmitters in the catecholamine system, for example, are reduced in some elderly brains. The catecholamines, which include dopamine (reduced in Parkinson's disease), epinephrine (the "fight or flight" hormone), and norepinephrine (reduced in depression), are also found in decreased amounts in the elderly. So is the neurotransmitter called GABA (short for gamma-amino-butyric acid), the major inhibitory transmitter in the brain. A decline in GABA could mean that brain cells begin firing randomly, leaving afterimages that take a longer time to fade. The clinical observation of a GABA deficiency could be considered evidence to support the "neural noise" hypothesis propounded in the 1950s to explain cognitive slowing with age. (We will learn more about the neural noise hypothesis in chapter 3.)

But not all neurotransmitters decline with age. Of the twenty-five proven or suspected transmitters, most remain at relatively constant levels in healthy old persons, and one, known as MAO (for monoamine oxidase), is thought to increase with age. "But MAO is a disaster," points out Lissy Jarvik, a professor at the University of California at Los Angeles and head of the psychogenetics unit at the Los Angeles Veterans Administration Hospital. "It's been linked to depression: the more MAO circulating, the more likely an individual is to be depressed." Still, some scientists believe that the increase in MAO is at least a hopeful sign, indicating that not everything about brain aging is a tale of inexorable loss. If MAO increases, perhaps some of the more useful neurotransmitters, such as the endorphins, may be found to increase with age, too. In fact, some studies of pain sensitivity have shown that old people have a better ability to mobilize the brain's morphine-like transmitter, beta-endorphin, and to use its pain-killing effect to best advantage. Whether because there's more beta-endorphin in storage in the aged brain, or because more is produced, or because the brain is simply more sensitive to the same amount, stimulation of the substance with a placebo, or inert, pill has been shown to reduce pain by 50 to 60 percent in old people. This result is almost as good as the 75 percent reduction of pain achieved with morphine injections, and much better than the 30 to 40 percent reduction achieved with placebo pills in the young.

The Old Brain's Paradox: Senile Plaques and Tangles

Which of the physical changes seen in the aged brain can be said to cause, directly or indirectly, changes in people's ability to think, react, learn, and remember as they get older? Therein lies the brain's paradox. The murkiness of the form-function relationship is particularly well illustrated in neuritic plaques and neurofibrillary tangles.

To learn the full story of these distinctive lesions of the brain, we must begin in the small English town of Newcastle-upon-Tyne, where three British pathologists, Blessed, Tomlinson, and Roth, began their comprehensive autopsy studies in the early 1960s. After studying the brains of seventy-eight elderly residents of the town, 36 percent of whom had died with none of the typical symptoms of "senility," the scientists made a remarkable discovery: More than 99 percent of the brains of people over the age of eighty showed signs of the brain lesions that had previously been associated only with a neurological disease known as pre-senile dementia. The lesions, called neurofibrillary tangles and neuritic plaques (or, sometimes, Alzheimer's plaques), were turning up not only in the brains of demented older people, but also in the brains of people who had functioned quite normally until the day they died. The only way to account for their abnormal-looking brains was by their age.

Blessed, Tomlinson, and Roth's findings suggest that formation of plaques and tangles in the brain is a part of normal aging (see chart). But these lesions have been blamed for the profound mental changes that accompany senile dementia, or Alzheimer's disease, because they occur in such great numbers in Alzheimer's patients. What, then, determines whether plaques and tangles will interfere with mental functioning? Why can some people have some lesions, or even a great deal of lesions, without losing their thinking powers, whereas others become "demented" even though their brains are relatively tangle-free and plaqueless?

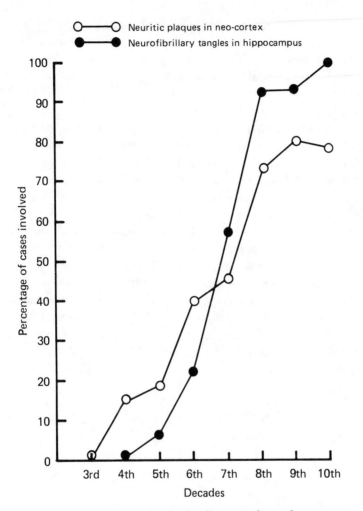

○────○ Neuritic plaques in neo-cortex
●────● Neurofibrillary tangles in hippocampus

3. Plaques and tangles in the general population.

According to Terry of the University of California at San Diego, the deciding factor is probably a matter of degree. Plaques and tangles "are present in small numbers in the functional elderly, and in large numbers in the senile," he says. "They seem to concentrate in direct proportion to the mental disability." The exceptions to this general rule of direct proportionality are just that—exceptions. And few scientists will venture a guess as to what makes these individuals different.

As the next chapter demonstrates, many of these physical changes in the aged brain are thought to account for a certain reduced mental capacity with age. The hallmarks of the aged intellect, according to many studies, are mild loss of memory and a somewhat slowed pace of intellectual functioning; and scientists have been able, with some degree of assurance, to attribute these changes to the physical changes just discussed. But mental decline is usually relatively mild in most old people and, in the absence of outright disease, doesn't appear until far into the seventies or even eighties. For most old people, then, the physical brain changes that occur with time usually do not translate directly into behavioral changes. In the next chapter, we investigate some of the non-anatomical factors that seem to make the difference.

3

Memory and Intelligence: How Much Is Lost?

"There is a wicked inclination in most people to suppose an old man decayed in his intellect," said the British scholar Samuel Johnson more than 200 years ago. "If a young or middle-aged man, when leaving a company, does not recollect where he laid his hat, it is nothing. But if the same inattention is discovered in an old man, people will shrug their shoulders and say 'His memory is going.' "

Some things have not changed much in 200 years: People still shrug their shoulders when an old man mislays his hat, and attribute it to the memory loss of age. They expect to see evidence of memory and intellectual decay in the elderly, and this expectation is usually transferred to the elderly themselves. Slips and oversights that might be ignored in youth strike terror in the hearts and minds of the aged. Is this the forgotten name, is this the lost key or forgotten purchase, that heralds the dreaded journey into the dark reaches of "senility"? How many more times can the eyeglasses be misplaced or the phone number misdialed before the more important thoughts and memories begin to crumble as well?

The prospect of intellectual functioning in the so-called twilight years is far more sunny than our folk tales would have it. Some changes in cognition (the mental operations through which we become aware of our surroundings, a process that includes thinking, perceiving, understanding, and reasoning) are a natural part of normal aging. Just as we wouldn't expect a seventy-five-year-old former athlete to run the mile as quickly as he could at twenty-five—even if he has stayed healthy and fit—we don't expect a seventy-five-year-old former professor to remain up-to-date in her field without a little extra effort, a little more time devoted to reading, studying, and writing. But the fact that the process is slower for her, the fact that she must now stop to look up citations that she could remember at will some forty years before, does not mean that she can no longer think, any more than the fact that the four-minute mile eludes the former runner means that he can no longer walk.

The myth about memory loss and intellectual decline with age is as powerful—and as destructive—as it is because the aged themselves have spent a lifetime believing it. We grow up expecting our grandparents, and then our parents, gradually to lose mental functioning, and as a result we treat them in ways that ensure that the myths will come true. When the time comes that we ourselves are defined as "old," we look for those same symptoms in ourselves.

"Society's prejudices indoctrinate us before they hit us," says Alex Comfort, the noted British gerontologist. "How many twenty-year-olds realize that sexual capacity and normal intelligence are lifelong in healthy humans? On this basis we obligingly drown ourselves as persons when the clock points to the appropriate age."

For most normal, healthy individuals, intellectual declines with age are relatively minor. The decline that does occur by and large revolves around one crucial function: speed. Aging is, in general, a time of slowing, slowing not only of gait and motor performance and metabolic processes but of certain intellectual and recall functions, too. In the absence of illness, though, most functions of the mind remain relatively intact. It's often our fear of mental infirmity, rather than an underlying biological process, that can turn a tendency to forget, a slacking of retentive power, into the very infirmity of which we're so afraid.

This chapter will look at some factors that account for the less profound changes of age: memory loss and intellectual slowing. The message is this: mental changes in normal, healthy aged adults are small and usually easily compensated for, and the few changes that do occur can be aggravated—indeed, may be created—by our expectation that old people are, by definition, less capable than they once were. To understand this, it is necessary to describe, first, the reasons for the intellectual changes of age, ranging from the sociological (many old people are assigned to nonroles in which thinking is unnecessary) to the psychological (a depressed individual, for example, functions less well than one who is not depressed) to the physiological (the changes in the brain, such as an increase in "neural noise" and a decrease of cells in the hippocampus). Then we will investigate some methods of minimizing even those few changes that do occur. Old dogs can be taught new tricks— and, if the tricks are taught correctly, can also remember them.

47

Forgetting: Benign or Malignant?

"Doctor, I can't seem to remember anything anymore," the seventy-three-year-old woman complained. "I go to the store, and I can't remember what I wanted to buy. I go out, and I can't remember whether I locked the door. I sit down to read, and I can't remember where I left my glasses. Sometimes I even forget what I had for breakfast that very morning."

Robert Kahn had seen many patients like this woman. A psychiatrist at the University of Chicago geriatric clinic, he had encountered hundreds of elderly people who complained of memory loss, especially memory for recent events. The complaints don't surprise him. "Why should she remember what she ate for breakfast?" he asks. "Her breakfasts are boring."

In 1974 Kahn conducted a study of 153 elderly persons, 113 of them psychiatric outpatients at the clinic and 40 of them members of the patients' families. About three-quarters of them (relatives and patients alike) complained of some memory loss; in more than 75 of them, the complaints were more than minimal. But, surprisingly, a test of objective memory revealed that, for healthy persons with no evidence of organic brain dysfunction, those who complained most bitterly about their memory problems had memories that worked perfectly well. The only explanation Kahn found for this memory complaint among healthy subjects was in a psychiatric test he also administered. The people who called themselves forgetful turned out to be, not forgetful, but depressed.

Depressed persons of any age have a weak self-image that is usually fed by stereotypes. When a teenager is depressed, he or she turns to the conventional notion of adolescence as a time of turmoil and rebelliousness; this explains why so-called juvenile delinquents often show high ratings for depression. In old age, the only available stereotype to which a depressed individual can turn is that of a forgetful old man or woman in "second childhood." When asked to describe their day-to-day functioning, depressed old people are likely to sigh and say, "It's not so good; I forget a lot." The emphasis in such a statement, though, is not on the forgetfulness; it's on the sadness.

"In addition to complaints about memory in general," Kahn reported in an article co-authored by Nancy Miller of the National Institute of Mental Health, "the depressed subjects showed a predilection for another common stereotype: that their memory for recent events was more impaired than their memory for remote events. When actually measured, it was found that there was no significant difference for memory of recent or remote events in any of the groups, and that those who complained about recent memory did as well as those who did not, but [the complainers] were significantly more depressed."

If it's not true, then why do so many people, both old and young, believe that recent memory fades sooner than remote memory? Kahn and Miller say the misunderstanding is due in part to the tests used to compare the two. On psychologists' tests of memory, they say, questions such as "When did World War II begin?" are asked to measure long-term memory. These answers are compared with answers to questions like "What did you have for breakfast yesterday?" that are asked to measure short-term memory. Thus, memory for events of global importance is compared with memory for events of personal insignificance. "We have sometimes suggested, with tongue in cheek, that it would be more comparable to test remote memory by asking, 'What did you have for breakfast on the morning of January 22, 1925?' " write Kahn and Miller. Another psychologist,

49

Jack Botwinick of Washington University, has suggested that if long-term memory does seem more intact in the aged, it may be because the memories we form at our most impressionable stage—between the ages of about fifteen and twenty-five—are the ones that stay with us most vividly for the rest of our lives.

The expectation of forgetfulness can haunt not only depressed individuals but also any older person. Kahn has seen it happen to some of his brightest colleagues at the University of Chicago. "Distinguished professors in their seventies who are still busily productive will complain about their memory impairment on the basis of such flimsy evidence as forgetting the name of the author of a paper," he says, "when they are still the same intensely preoccupied, absentminded persons they have always been."

Absentmindedness is merely amusing—and, at worst, inconvenient—in a forty-year-old. At seventy, it can be devastating, unless one remembers that forgetfulness in old age is in fact no more harmful, and only slightly more inconvenient, than it was in middle age. "I have long believed that the best way to remember to take something with me is to put it on the doorstep, so I can see it when I leave," says one seventy-four-year-old. "Now this works better if the object is big enough to trip me."

Gerontologists today distinguish between two kinds of forgetfulness: benign and malignant. "Benign forgetfulness is when you spend fifteen minutes looking for the glasses you mislaid," says Richard Besdine of the Harvard Medical School. "Malignant forgetfulness is when you forget you ever had glasses."

Benign forgetfulness is as common in old age as it was in youth; the difference is that in the elderly it can easily be turned into malignant forgetfulness by a culture that moves by too quickly, denying the aged the time they need to remember. One hint of how many old people at least worry about their memories is in the response to an advertisement that ran in the *New York Times* from 1976 to 1983. "Poor Memory or Depression?" read the ad. "Persons 60–85 years of age with mild to moderately severe symptoms of poor memory, or with moderate to severe depression, may qualify to volunteer for programs with new medication." Some 600 persons a year responded to the ad, (which was dropped in 1983 because word-of-mouth advertising brought volunteers enough); approximately one-third of them had memory loss considered perfectly normal for their age.

"When I go down to my boat, I have to go over and over in my head the night before what I want to take along with me," said one man, aged sixty-nine, who answered the advertisement, placed by the Geriatric Study Program at New York University. "I think, 'I want to take my electric drill, and two pieces of mahogany of this length and this width, and a box of nails.' But when I go to the boat the next morning, I get all the way there before I realize I forgot the drill!"

The severity of this kind of forgetfulness is a very subjective matter. In this man's case, his memory lapses may have seemed harmless enough to an outsider, since he was still able to sail, teach a navigation course, operate a ham radio, and read voraciously. But inside his head, the memory loss was distressing. "I love to learn," he said. "Now I have trouble retaining things." His new forgetfulness was responsible, he thought, for his difficulty in obtaining a higher class of ham operator license.

Another man who answered the same ad described his forgetfulness this way: "Every evening, I would unload all the junk from my pants pocket and put it on the dresser in the bedroom. Every morning, I would get dressed and put the things back in my pocket. But when I got downstairs to the kitchen, it always turned out I had forgotten something up in the bedroom." After four months of therapy at the New York University clinic—including an experimental trial of the drug L-dopa and frequent return visits for on-going memory tests—this man, aged seventy-three, felt his memory was improving. "Now I only have to get halfway down the stairs before I remember that I forgot."

With his graphic illustration, this man has unwittingly provided a useful model for the memory process—and the way in which the process is impaired with age. When young people forget something, the lapse between forget-ting and remembering that they forgot is usually small. At worst, a businessman may remember at 1:30 P.M. that he had a lunch appointment at noon, or a person may recall late in the day that she had meant to stop at the dry cleaner's on her way in to work. For the elderly, though, the recall may take days to surface.

Were it not for the social and psychological stresses of being old in contemporary America, this irksome slowness rarely would turn into the more flagrant memory loss of malignant forgetfulness. Even in this less-than-perfect world, most old people manage to get along with their be-nign memory losses. Among persons over age eighty—virtu-ally all of whom are presumed to encounter some diffi-culty with memory—only a fraction, ranging in estimates from 10 to 30 percent of the very old, experience profound loss of memory.

Several factors, though, can help turn benign forgetful-ness into malignant forgetfulness. Depression is one—a pessimistic view of oneself and the world that exaggerates small failings into big disabilities. Fear can do the same thing, touching off what one social worker calls "the spiral of senility." In this configuration, forgetfulness creates anx-iety, which in turn creates, in tragic succession, depen-dence, more forgetfulness, more fear and anxiety, and finally the kind of confused, withdrawn behavior that leads to the categorization of "senility."

Another enemy of the forgetful elderly, a factor that can turn memory loss from benign to malignant, is boredom. In a society that has no time, no place, no role for old people, the elderly have little chance to use and exercise their minds. When one aimless day blends into the next, when it does not seem to matter whether it's Tuesday or Wednesday, why bother to keep track? When one's breakfasts and lunches are the only change in routine, and even they are too bland to recall, why bother to remember? When well-meaning friends and relatives help out with the laundry, the finances, the shopping, the cleaning, so that the chores of everyday life require no thought or mental exertion, why bother to pay attention? If the mind isn't used it goes blank, and if nothing new is put into the memory store — an activity that requires some effort and concentration — then the well is dry when one tries to remember. Persons who have lost the habit of thinking, of recalling, have trouble each time they make the attempt, and the delay and difficulty feed their frustration and make them even more reticent to try the next time.

Boredom, fear, and depression are able to influence memory because the process itself is so fragile. Memory, it seems, is not simply cellular or biochemical or electrical or genetic in nature. It is instead an amalgam of all these processes in the brain. And psychologists have found that one's overall mind-set, encompassing such idiosyncrasies as motivation, attention span, concentration, and competitiveness, as well as one's physical health, are involved in one's ability to remember. Thus, the frequent observation that old people lose their memory, especially their memory for recent events, may well have its origin in a characteristic that has nothing to do with age.

The Routes of Recall

It is hard to draw a map of just what paths an impulse travels before it is stored away in the "memory warehouse" of the brain. But experimental psychologists and neuroscientists are at least developing some idea today of which brain structures and components are important in the process of memory formation, storage, and retrieval. They know, for example, that the central memory region is probably the hippocampus of the brain, where memory seems to be readied for storage; that RNA is probably involved in memory formation, perhaps by being manufactured in a specific way to correspond to an item learned and remembered; that the cholinergic system is vital to memory, since animals and humans in whom these neurotransmitters are deficient have been rendered amnesic; and that an adequate complement of neurons in the frontal cortex is needed to receive the messages that pass through on their way to longer-term storage.

Gerontologists still don't know how much memory loss is inherent in the aging process. Older test subjects perform consistently less well than younger subjects on psychological tests of memory, even when the results are corrected for such confounding factors as health, motivation, and speed. But that fact alone need not mean that memory loss is a part of normal aging—any more than the fact that most old people have fat deposits in their blood vessels means that atherosclerosis is a part of normal aging. Atherosclerosis, we now know, is a disease probably brought on by a lifetime of poor eating and exercise habits coupled with a genetic predisposition to blood vessel clogging. Can it be that the same can be said for the forgetfulness of age?

"We have all been taught that 'the brain is not a muscle' that can be maintained, the way the heart can, through exercise," notes geriatric psychologist Lissy Jarvik of the University of California at Los Angeles. "When it comes to the effects of inactivity, however, perhaps the brain is like a muscle after all." Jarvik bases her conclusion on a detailed longitudinal (life-long) study of aged twins, begun in upstate New York in the late 1940s. Twin studies, though cumbersome to conduct, are invaluable to psychologists interested in separating genetic effects (which can be held constant within identical twin pairs, whose similarities are then compared with those of non-identical twins) from the effects of the environment. Nearly thirty years after her study of 134 sets of aged twins began, Jarvik found that "continued mental activity, even more so than physical activity," characterized the twins who aged most successfully. "Persons who engaged in cognitive, emotive, and physical activities on a regular basis throughout adulthood aged more successfully than those who were relatively inactive," she said. And it's never too late to rouse yourself from your rocking chair: "Activities in later life, rather than those of earlier years, were primarily related to successful aging."

Jarvik's twin study is among the dozen or so longitudinal studies conducted over the last quarter-century to discover to what extent mental changes may be considered a normal part of aging. Most of these studies have revealed far fewer mental losses, and losses occurring at much later ages, than had been expected based on the myth of decline that was popular in the 1940s and 1950s. Yet even these optimistic results do reveal some decline on certain test scores with age. The question then arises: Do the normal physical changes seen in the healthy aged brain explain a general, expected decline, however slight, in one's ability to think and to remember? If the brain structures involved in recall—be it a memory center, components of neural circuitry, certain neurotransmitters, or the genetic compound RNA—inevitably change somewhat with age, do these biological changes eventually reveal themselves in at least some mental decline, no matter how healthy and active a seventy- or eighty-year-old might be?

As we look for answers, we must bear in mind that this simplification of the issue does an injustice, as do most simplifications, to the intricacies of memory function in the elderly. "At any age, memory is a complex phenomenon, subject to the effects of non-cognitive factors such as personality and motivation," write Kahn and Miller. "But in the aged, especially, memory function is more than the reflection of a cognitive deficit based on structural brain changes. . . . [Sometimes] memory 'impairment' represents adaptive behavior related to depression, stress, and/or noxious environments, and can thus be prevented, modified, or reversed."

In their efforts to discover which memory changes are a part of aging per se and which are created by "depression, stress and/or noxious environments," some scientists are turning to animal models. Laboratory animals are not subject to the effects of expectations of memory loss, of the spiral of senility, or of the particular hazards of being old in Western society. Laboratory animals do not, as people may, lose their memories in reaction to intolerable life situations, or as a result of such stresses as relocation or retirement.

Animal Memory and Choline

One study by Raymond T. Bartus is instructive in this regard. Bartus and his colleagues at the Parke-Davis Research Laboratory compared the short-term memory of young and old rhesus monkeys. In order to avoid the possible confusing effects of age-related differences in psychomotor coordination, motivation, attention, or visual acuity, Bartus used an automated contraption that the monkeys learned to maneuver at their own pace. This made Bartus sure that what he was measuring was the effect of age itself on memory. He found that age, at least in rhesus monkeys, seems to cause a definite decline in the animal's ability to retain information. "The deficit was so large," he said, "that there existed no overlap at all in performance between groups." In other words, even the *best* memory scores for the older monkeys (aged eighteen to twenty-one, or approximately seventy to seventy-five in human years) were still lower than the *worst* scores for the younger monkeys (who were three or four years old, or about fifteen in human years). The difference, he said, can be attributed to "a specific deficit in short-term memory [that] does occur as a consequence of the aging process."

Reflecting his pharmaceutical bent, Bartus explained his findings in light of biochemical changes in the aged brain, specifically the observed decrease in neurotransmitters in the cholinergic system. "The nature of this [memory] deficit [in the older monkeys] bears a striking resemblance to that produced in [younger] monkeys when tested in this exact same procedure under low doses of the anticholinergic scopolamine," he said. Scopolamine reduces the brain level of the neurotransmitter acetylcholine. Thus, it mimics the chemical situation of the typical aged brain, since the amount of available acetylcholine is significantly reduced, perhaps by as much as 70 percent, in the brains of people in their seventies or eighties.

If monkeys whose acetylcholine is artificially reduced perform identically to monkeys who are simply old—and therefore, presumably, also suffering a relative deficit of acetylcholine—perhaps stimulation of this neurotransmitter can help minimize the memory losses of age, Bartus reasoned. This theory is offered here only as a possible explanation for the observed benign forgetfulness of older people; in chapter 7 we will return to clinical studies that have been undertaken to see whether the administration of choline or related chemicals seems to improve memory in the aged. (A preview: The results so far are disappointing.)

Memory and the Hippocampus

Another explanation for the memory loss of old age could lie within the hippocampus. This twisted configuration of neurons, tucked under the side lobes of the cerebral cortex and named the Greek word for "sea horse" to describe its shape, is widely thought to be the memory center of the brain. All events are thought to enter the brain first through the hippocampus, where they are processed for storage into long-term memory. The mechanism of storage may be a biochemical change in the brain, an alteration of genetic material there, synthesis of a new protein, or imprinting of a new groove of neural circuitry. Those events that are not somehow translated into permanent form are relegated to a short-term memory bank from which the image will eventually fade.

The importance of the hippocampus in memory processing is graphically documented in the case of one gruesome living experiment, a man known in the medical literature as Henry M. Beginning in his childhood, Henry had experienced frequent epileptic seizures; by the time he was twenty-seven they had become so severe that he was forced to quit work, and his doctor was prepared to take drastic measures. This was in the 1950s, when neurosurgeons were successfully treating epilepsy by removing one lobe of the hippocampus. Since Henry's seizures were so severe and widespread, his surgeon, S. B. Scoville, decided to remove both hippocampal lobes.

Scoville apparently was unaware that the hippocampus is the seat of all recent memory, the place where impressions are received in order to be processed, stored, and later retrieved by other brain structures. Since his operation in 1953, Henry M. has been unable to remember anything.

The Canadian scientist Brenda Milner has spent countless hours working with Henry at the Montreal Neurological Institute. He never recognizes her. He has no knowledge of the date, the year, his own age, his family's address, the tasks he's done before. He works on the same jigsaw puzzle again and again, reads the same magazines without knowledge of ever having seen them. Ironically, he can "learn" motor skills as easily as normal subjects, and performs well at his job on an assembly line. But he has no conscious recollection of the task from day to day, and can't even remember that he has a job. Although his scores on lab tests of motor performance invariably improve with repetition—an indication of a kind of "learning"—Henry cannot recall having done the tests before. Without a hippocampus, he has no place to lay down his memories, and thus no store from which to retrieve them. "Right now, I'm wondering, have I done or said anything amiss?" he once confessed. "You see, at this moment everything looks clear to me, but what happened just before? That's what worries me. . . . Every day is alone in itself, whatever enjoyment I've had, and whatever sorrow I've had."

If Henry concentrates hard enough, he is able to remember, after a fashion; but the effort he must expend, and the total disappearance of the memory once he stops concentrating, are tragic. As Milner describes it:

He was able to retain the number 584 for at least 15 minutes,
by continuously working out elaborate mnemonic schemes.
When asked how he had been able to retain the number for
so long, he replied: "It's easy. You just remember 8. You see,
5, 8, and 4 add to 17. You remember 8, subtract it from 17
and it leaves 9. Divide 9 in half and you get 5 and 4, and
there you are: 584. Easy!" A minute or so later [Henry] was
unable to recall either the number 584 or any of the associ-
ated complex train of thought; in fact, he did not know that
he had been given a number to remember because in the
meantime the examiner had introduced a new topic.

In a profoundly exaggerated way, Henry's condition
resembles the state of the aged brain. The hippocampus is
thought by many scientists to lose as much as 40 percent
of its cells by the time an individual reaches his eighties.
More important even than the loss of cells, though, is the
loss that occurs in arborization, or branching out, of the
dendrite network in the hippocampus. As we saw in chapter 2, Madge and Arnold Scheibel and their co-workers at
UCLA's Institute for Brain Research found that the intricate dendritic branches in this part of the brain are shorn of
as many as 60 to 80 percent of their filaments by the age of
about eighty or ninety. These dendrites are essential for
conducting both impulses and nutrients within the neuron
and from one neuron to another; without them, in short,
the neuron cannot do its work. It remains to be tested how
much this decline of arborization in the hippocampus can
be linked to a corresponding decline in intellectual and
memory functioning among old people.

Closely related to its role as the seat of incoming memory is the hippocampus's function as the brain's adventure
seeker. From an evolutionary perspective, this dual role
makes sense: In order to survive in the wild, an animal
must evolve both the capacity to remember where it has
been and the urge to explore places yet unseen. The hip-

pocampus reflects this urge for novelty in two ways. It stimulates us to search out whatever is new, as can be seen in the behavior of experimental animals whose hippocampi have been surgically removed: they exhibit none of the zest for exploration shown by their intact peers. And just as the hippocampus stimulates novelty, novelty stimulates the hippocampus. Hippocampal cells give off only minimal indications of activity, as measured on the electroencephalogram (EEG), when laboratory animals are immobile. Brain activity increases when the animals move about, and increases even more when the animals are in the throes of discovery. The analogy between the motionless, caged animals and old people, themselves rendered immobile due to physical, social, or economic constraints, is hard to resist. If the hippocampus of the aged brain finds nothing novel in its environment to keep it fired up, is it any wonder that when it is called on to produce a remembered image, it often hasn't the reserve power to do so?

Memory and Neural Noise

Another theory as to why memory function may decline over a lifetime is the generally overlooked, but nonetheless intriguing, "neural noise" hypothesis. This point of view, most forcefully expressed by several British scientists in the late 1950s, suggests that old brains are riddled with a high level of background noise, with which incoming impulses must compete if they are to be recognized, selected out, and acted upon. This background noise, the theory goes, may be due to one of several observed brain changes with age: the slower rate at which neural impulses subside, which means that traces of previous stimulations hover for much longer than they do in the young; a loss of healthy, active neurons, which ordinarily would smooth over the effect of occasional random firings from abnormal neurons; or, as we discussed in chapter 2, a general increase in the level of brain sensitivity, adopted in response to the reduced overall receptiveness of the aged brain, but resulting also in a distractingly high level of background noise.

Whatever the origin of the noisy brain, its effect, in the words of psychologist A. T. Welford, is thought to be as follows: "A signal represents a rise of activity above the ambient level. Since, however, the [background] level fluctuates, a signal must be 'sampled' for an appreciable time if it is to be distinguished reliably from the background 'noise,' and the length of sample needed will depend on the signal-to-noise ratio, becoming longer as the signal becomes weaker or as the 'noise' increases." In short, the neural noise would lead to mental slowing, as the individual takes longer and longer to figure out which impulses are new and important and which are part of the general hum that is always there.

As Welford points out, this hypothesis is "neurologically crude," but it provides a helpful model for the mechanism that might bring into play a range of psychological, psychomotor, and neurological factors. Its great advantage is that it highlights the one overriding characteristic of age, the factor that has become notorious in its confounding of classic tests of memory and intelligence in older subjects: the factor of speed.

A Matter of Time

The world rushed past her. She couldn't concentrate and was failing miserably at even the simplest tasks. What happened to the time when things had moved at her pace? Her thoughts were racing, and her body ached. Why were her hands moving so slowly? Why did her mind creak so? Frustrated by her frequent mistakes, angry at herself for forgetting so many details, she finally gave up, grumbling.

A crotchety old woman, long past her prime, obviously forgetful, rigid—senile? No, this was a young college student participating in a classroom psychology experiment conducted by Dr. Robert Kastenbaum at Wayne State University. In order to demonstrate the behavioral impact that just one lone trait—slowness—can have in the elderly, Kastenbaum invented a game in which a speeded-up environment created an aura he called "pre-experiencing age."

The thirty-one students involved in Kastenbaum's experiment were between the ages of eighteen and twenty-four. Each was assigned the task of "rebuilding" a mock village supposedly shattered by war. Two sets of file cards were presented—one set describing the jobs that needed to be done, the other describing the available people to do them—and each student was told to match each job with the best-suited individual. There were about 100 job cards and 150 manpower cards to manipulate. At first, Kastenbaum allowed each student five minutes to match a job card with a manpower card, and a bell signaled when it was time to move on to the next job card. Without the subjects knowing it, though, he gradually stepped up the pace of the experiment, ringing the bell every four minutes, then three, then two. As the tempo quickened, these young students began to "act old." Indeed, by the time the bell was ringing at twice its original frequency, they were virtually paralyzed in their decision making.

"The students began to engage in random actions—picking up a card, putting it down, picking it up again," Kastenbaum says. "Some narrowed their focus and kept working with the same few cards. Some became almost stultified, some jittery and agitated. Even though many of them were aware that we were speeding things along, they still took it out on themselves when they couldn't perform fast enough. They were angry at themselves, angry that what had started out as a manageable task had become so complicated."

As this study shows, when things move too quickly, one's performance—and, just as important, one's motivation—drops precipitously. This small truth has been revealed to psychologists only in the last decade or so, and has forced them to reappraise all of the cognitive performance test scores that have, over the years, contributed to the notion that memory and intelligence decline with age. What, they are asking now, were those earlier experiments really testing? Sometimes, it seems, they were tapping not into memory or intelligence itself, but into quick memory and ready intelligence. They were testing, too, the aged subjects' ability to perform under the test conditions of the laboratory, rather than their ability to compensate for their mild losses and to function independently in the community.

The effect of slowing on memory in the aged was graphically illustrated in studies conducted in the early 1970s by psychologist T. R. Anders. Anders found that the "rate of search"—the pace at which an individual can sift through his memory roster to come up with the correct bit of information on demand—is significantly reduced with age. As Alex Comfort has described it, "the index file doesn't age, but the secretary is older and takes longer to put new cards in or to bring cards you want." The memory, in other words, is still there, still tucked away somewhere; but older people, for a host of physical and perhaps psychological reasons, just take longer finding it.

Anders confirmed this index card analogy in his rate-of-search studies. He presented number lists of varying lengths to three groups of people, aged nineteen to twenty-one, thirty-three to forty-three, and fifty-eight to eighty-five. The subjects were asked to memorize the numbers on each list, and then to respond "yes" or "no" to flash cards of digits presented one at a time—"yes" if the number on the card had appeared on the memorized list, "no" if it hadn't. Taking for granted that the answer was correct, Anders recorded only the speed of response. This, he reasoned, was a measure of how long it took to search the store of short-term memory—the list of numbers—and to retrieve the correct information.

As the length of the list grew, from one number to three to five to seven, all age groups took longer to say "yes" or "no" when confronted with a flash card. But the additional digits slowed down the middle-aged and old groups more than they slowed down the young subjects. Anders concluded that, beginning in middle age, the rate of search diminishes, and this slowing down becomes progressively more detrimental as one must search an ever-larger memory store.

If older people are allowed more time to perform on certain memory and intelligence tests, then, are they able to do as well as younger people do? The answer, generally, is yes. Test after test designed in a self-paced mode, or reinterpreted to eliminate the confounding factors of speed, show that many memory functions and most intelligence functions remain intact far into the ninth decade in healthy old folks. Indeed, some intelligence test scores, such as vocabulary—a skill that requires an intact memory as well as a full store of knowledge—are shown on self-paced tests to increase with age.

This new consensus has been encouraging for elderly people concerned about their mental prowess. If society just learns to slow things down a little, this approach tells us, and to wait for its parents and grandparents until they have had sufficient time to think and remember, we will find that old people are as bright as they ever were, and in many respects even brighter. But this positive outlook must be tempered with one nagging question: In dismissing the factor of speed when we look at test performance on measures of memory and intelligence, are we in fact dismissing the very quality we mean when we speak of intelligence, the very quality that makes a person "smart"?

Psychologist James Birren of the University of Southern California, though a long-time advocate of the elderly and a believer in the lifelong maintenance of intelligence, suspects that speed may be central to the mental processes we are now saying remain relatively intact in old age *except* for speed. Speed is not peripheral in matters of the mind, he suggests; it is what distinguishes the capable from the less capable. Thus, it may be invalid to parcel out speed in an attempt to assess mental skills without it.

Take memory, for instance. It may be that too great a slowing down in the process of memory finally obliterates the memory forever. "Given a rapid decay system in memory [at any age]," Birren says, "a sluggishness in processing information would preclude the opportunity of using decaying information in combination with other stimuli. In brief, I suggest that man is not simply a calculator that is slowing down because of an electrical brownout [an image many have used to describe the effect on mental processes of the slowing down of age], but man is a calculator that has some components that decay with time. . . . If the events are not completed within a time limit, the possibility of the task being completed successfully is diminished."

Aging means an essential slowing of information processing, Birren says. "If there is a central slowing of processing or mediation, then all phenomena we regard as important in behavior will slow down. Perception and memory will become less efficient, as will retrieval from the long-term store of previously learned material. Furthermore, the likelihood of novel associations will decrease."

Recall vs. Recognition

With this caveat in mind, let us explore some other psychological test findings that give clues as to the way in which memory functions change with age. Even while recognizing, as Birren does, that speed is a central, not an incidental, part of thought and memory, we can nonetheless find studies that confirm the conviction that most memory loss is benign, and that most old people keep their wits about them far into the "twilight years."

One way to obtain evidence for this optimistic outlook is to divide the process of memory into separate components, and then to determine which part of the process is affected by age. When an item is "learned" (that is, remembered), it is processed and stored; when it is needed again, the memory of the item is retrieved from storage. Where along the line of processing, storage, and retrieval does the greatest age-related change occur?

Once again, the experts are split. But a growing consensus seems to be that old people suffer most in the process of retrieval—and that's good news for the elderly. "If the problem is storage," notes psychologist Jack Botwinick, "the [information] is forgotten and can never be recalled. The information is no longer available. If the problem is retrieval and not storage, then the information is available but not accessible." This latter situation is far to be preferred, since old people can be taught devices for calling up the stored information. Alex Comfort's aged "secretary" can simply be given a refresher course in how to search through the index file more effectively — and this can work so long as the index cards have not been written on with vanishing ink.

Among the studies that indicate that retrieval, not storage, is the function that declines with age, the Canadian scientist David Schonfield's is one of the most informative. Schonfield designed his study to differentiate between two types of memory: recall, or the memory involved in answering the question "What was the name of your high school English teacher?"; and recognition, such as is involved in answering the same question posed as "Does one of these names sound familiar?" Schonfield theorized that recall would tap the viability of the storage mechanism, and recognition would measure retrieval.

The test worked this way: A group of subjects, ranging in age from twenty to seventy-five, was asked to recite a list of twenty-four words they had committed to memory. This recitation was designed to test recall ability, a measure of the storage function. To test recognition, which reflects retrieval skills, Schonfield had the subjects memorize a second list of twenty-four words, and then gave them clues when he asked them to call up those words from memory. He administered a test composed of twenty-four questions, each of which consisted of five words: four new words, and one selected from the memorized list. The test subjects had to circle the words they had seen before.

Schonfield's results (summarized in the chart that follows) show that only one kind of memory was impaired with age: recall. In fact, recognition scores actually improved among the old subjects. If older people seem to have trouble with memory, he concluded, it's because the secretary doesn't move about as quickly as she used to—not because the information is no longer in the file.

Sometimes, though, the information may be there somewhere, but it's nearly impossible to find because it's filed in the wrong place. In these instances, the secretary is showing her age in a different way: trained in the old school where filing was by the alphabet, she just cannot understand the logic of the new office's system of filing by conceptual category—or, worse yet, by computer code number.

These mistakes in "storage" functions of memory are more profound than the sluggishness of "retrieval." If information is stored in the wrong place, the process of retrieving it becomes interminable. Many psychologists believe

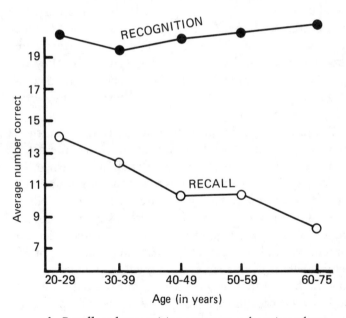

4. *Recall and recognition scores as a function of age.*

that these mistakes are not inherent in the aging process itself, but are usually the result of an educational or training deficit that puts old people at a disadvantage in their effort to store and learn new information in the first place.

The process of storing new information, or learning, involves such mental gymnastics as categorization, integration, and patterning—skills that were not taught in the learning-by-rote schools that most of today's elderly attended. Thus, initial learning in the aged is far short of what learning is for the younger generation. And old people, just like young people, cannot remember what they have never learned.

This truism was brought home in a classic study conducted by psychologists S. H. Davis and Walter Obrist. They studied two groups of adults—aged nineteen to thirty-five and sixty-five to eighty-four—who were matched according to intellectual ability, and had each group learn a list of paired words. Two minutes later, the subjects were asked to recall the list, and in forty-eight hours they returned to the lab for another retest. Thus each group compiled three scores: for initial learning, short-term memory, and long-term memory.

The older group performed consistently less well than the younger group. But Davis and Obrist were interested not in learning but in retention of what was learned, so they adjusted the memory scores to account for age-related differences in initial learning scores. And, *voilá!* When these adjustments were made, the groups showed no difference in their forty-eight-hour retention of what had been learned. Not only did this show that old people cannot remember what they have never learned, but—more important—it showed that they *could* remember what they *had* learned. As succeeding generations of the aged become better educated and more conversant with efficient methods of learning, the observed fall-off in memory with age may become even less apparent.

In the meantime, today's elderly—with an average educational level of the eighth grade and a general inability to catch on to such concept-based learning skills as "the new math"—are indeed handicapped when it comes to abstract thinking and other mental skills needed in our high-technology world. This relative deficit reflects not a decline but a difference in early educational and life experiences. It has contributed, nonetheless, to the perpetuation of another myth about the mental changes of age: the myth of declining intelligence.

Intelligence: Must What Goes Up Come Down?

Like attic walls, the aged brain gathers dust and cobwebs only when it is not in use. But for most people, thought remains an integral part of daily life far into old age. Unlike forgetfulness, which is probably to be expected—in its benign form—in most old people, a decline in intellectual functioning need not occur with the passage of the years. Far more important than chronological age itself are other factors, many of them associated with extreme old age, that predict a good deal about performance on intelligence tests: physical health, early educational experiences, and distance from death.

The myth of sliding intelligence developed out of a series of carefully designed studies conducted in the first half of this century—carefully designed but wrongheaded. Old volunteers were given intelligence tests, the most popular being the Wechsler Adult Intelligence Scale developed in 1955 to remove the cultural biases found in the traditional Stanford-Binet intelligence test. Their scores were then compared with the scores of young volunteers. The younger subjects always did better.

These cross-sectional studies, which looked at various age groups of the population at a fixed point in time, conspired to create the scientific impression that intellectual functioning increased into young adulthood, plateaued during the twenties and thirties, and began a slow and steady decline at about age forty. As psychologists Paul Baltes and K. Warner Schaie have observed, "the textbook view coincided with the everyday notion that, as far as intelligence is concerned, what goes up must come down."

Baltes and Schaie were among the first to challenge that notion. They did so with longitudinal studies—studies that follow a particular group of people over a long period of time, and thus deny younger groups the unfair advantage they usually have on intelligence tests because of their superior health and education. In 1956 Schaie selected 500 subjects, ranging in age from twenty-one to seventy, and gave them two tests of cognitive function—Thurstone's Primary Mental Abilities Test and his own Test of Behavioral Rigidity. Seven years later, 301 of the original 500 subjects returned to take the same two tests again.

"If we analyze the data cross-sectionally (comparing the different age groups at a given point in time), we see the conventional pattern of early, systematic decline," Schaie reports. "But when we look at the results longitudinally (comparing a given age group's performance in 1956 with its performance in 1963), we find a definite decline on only one of the four measures, visuo-motor flexibility," and a systematic increase in the most important dimension of mental ability, crystallized intelligence. The improvement in this measure, which reflects such abilities as verbal comprehension, numerical skills, and inductive reasoning, continued "right into old age. Even people over seventy improved from the first testing to the second."

As shown in the chart on page 74, the method of comparison makes all the difference. Why does a cross-sectional interpretation of the data show a marked decline with age, while a longitudinal interpretation not only shows no decline but sometimes shows an increase? Scientists account for the discrepancy with what they call the "cohort factor." Consider the difference in life experiences, culture, education, career patterns, in two women of equal intelligence born fifteen years apart: 1910 versus 1925, for example, or 1940 versus 1955. Younger subjects, who tend to be better-educated, more schooled in test taking, and more likely to have lived a life of relative ease and opportunity, almost invariably score better than older subjects. The differences in scores is due, not to the biological effects of age, but to the differences in thinking and performing style from one generation to another.

Several factors confound the results of cross-sectional tests. Motivation differs between young and old. Older people simply don't care quite as much about making an impressive display. Old people also have been shown to exhibit more caution than the young, waiting until they're absolutely certain before venturing an answer—a trait that can significantly lower test scores when points are not deducted for guessing. And perhaps most important is the factor of speed. As we have seen, speed at recall and performance is one of the most obvious losses that accompany age, and most intelligence tests are time-bound—thus requiring a skill at which the young excel. Once again, though, we must remember James Birren's nagging question: Which is a "more valid indicator of that elusive quality we call intelligence," an intelligence test taken with time constraints or one taken without them?

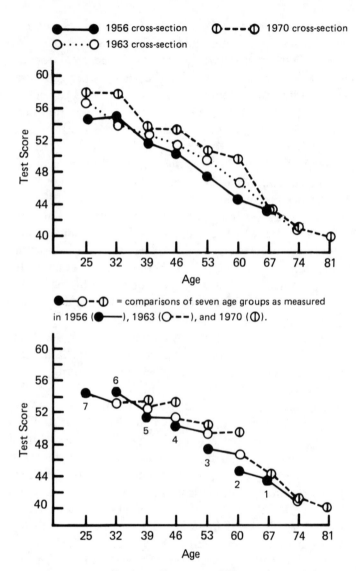

5. *Differences in fluid intelligence (problem-solving ability) with age as measured by a) cross-sectional studies and b)longitudinal studies.*

In Sickness or in Health?

But speed, motivation, and the "cohort factor" do not account for all the differences observed between young and old on tests of intelligence. Some longitudinal studies have found that declines in intelligence scores are associated with physical conditions that become more and more frequent with age: hypertension, disorders of the immune system, chromosome loss, and, perhaps most dramatically, nearness to death.

Carl Eisdorfer, when he was at the University of Washington, was among the first to relate hypertension (high blood pressure) to a fall-off of intellectual power with age. He and his colleagues gave intelligence tests to two groups of older people—people in their sixties and people in their seventies—and gave them the same tests ten years later. When the subjects were divided according to their diastolic blood pressure into normal pressure (66-95 for the "bottom" reading of blood pressure), mildly elevated pressure (96–105), and high pressure (over 105), a significant difference in their scores over time was revealed—especially for those persons who were aged sixty to sixty-nine when the testing began. In this younger group, the greatest fall-off in performance was noted in the high blood pressure group, and the normal pressure group showed only a mild decline in performance. Interestingly, the group with mildly elevated blood pressure actually improved between the first intelligence test and the second. (All these changes were recorded for the nonverbal subtests of the Wechsler Adult Intelligence Scale, which have been found to be most sensitive to age-related changes. The subtests for verbal intelligence showed no significant decline in any of the groups).

Eisdorfer hypothesized that mild blood pressure elevation may protect old people from intellectual slowing, since it assures that the brain receives a sufficient supply of blood. This protective effect, however, was lost in the older group of test subjects, who were in their seventies when Eisdorfer began his study and in their eighties when they were retested. For this group, results were more difficult to interpret, since everyone in the high blood pressure group had died before the second test.

Merrill Elias, a psychologist at the University of Maine at Orono, disagrees with Eisdorfer's findings. "There is no evidence that uncomplicated hypertensives are brain damaged or show intellectual deficits," he says. "The differences between hypertensive and normotensive samples may reflect subject selection variables and other unknown and [as] yet uncontrolled factors, such as drug taking or the presence of hypertension-related complications."

Other longitudinal studies add weight to the general scientific impression that health status, not age per se, is the most important determinant of whether one will experience some fall-off in intelligence. The immune system, which protects the body from invading organisms, has been shown to go through such marked decline with age that some scientists have wondered whether aging itself is an immune disease. The theory of auto-immunity, in which the body's defense mechanisms are turned upon itself, has been proposed to explain certain age-related losses, including the loss of brain cells. Kalidas Nandy of Boston University, for example, found anti-brain antibodies in the bloodstream of old mice but not of young mice, and showed that these antibodies are capable of slowly permeating the blood-brain barrier and perhaps causing "scattered loss of nerve cells in the brain of old animals." In humans, research is just beginning that links auto-immune diseases with declines in performance on intelligence tests.

Like hypertension and immune diseases, chromosome loss is another physical problem that occurs more frequently with age—and that has been linked to a general decline in intelligence. All cells in the body have forty-six chromosomes—twenty-three pairs—but occasionally, with increasing age, some cells are detected with only forty-four or forty-five. This is especially true in older women, leading some investigators to conclude that the chromosome loss may be due to a problem of replication in the X chromosome, while the Y chromosome remains intact. (Of the twenty-three chromosome pairs, one is the pair coding for sex: two X chromosomes in females, and one X chromosome and one Y chromosome in males.)

At birth, only 3.5 percent of the cells in the body are missing a chromosome, a relatively harmless anomaly that usually has few behavioral or health effects. But by the age of sixty-five, women encounter an incidence of chromosome loss as high as 9.5 to 12.8 percent. At this rate, the loss of chromosomes, called hypodiploidy, may have significant behavioral effects.

Several additional studies have given weight to the hypothesis that chromosome loss is related to cognitive change. The Danish scientist Johannes Nielsen found a significant incidence of hypodiploidy—16.9 percent—in a group of elderly women hospitalized with senile dementia, compared to only 10.1 percent incidence of chromosome loss in normal women of the same age, and just 3.9 percent in women below the age of forty. Lissy Jarvik of the University of California at Los Angeles has found that chromosome loss in older women is correlated with poor performance on psychological and cognitive tests, especially tests of visual memory and cognitive development. Jarvik admits to puzzlement over the cause-and-effect relationship between chromosome loss and intellectual decline.

"Does the loss of chromosomes in glial cells of the brain . . . either directly or indirectly (by interfering with neuronal functioning) interfere with mental functioning?" she asks. "Or does the loss of chromosomes result in certain immunological changes that then also influence mental functioning? . . . Is chromosome loss perhaps not exclusively detrimental but also beneficial? Is it possible, for example, that a loss of chromosomes may protect to some extent against abnormal immune developments that characterize advancing age—the less chromosomal material subject to error, the fewer errors?" She offers no answers to these questions, but their persistence highlights the dangers involved in drawing hasty conclusions about the relationship between physical and mental events—particularly in the aged.

The Terminal Drop Hypothesis

The most dramatic example of this danger, at least in the study of aging and intelligence, is the terminal drop hypothesis. According to this theory, persons who show a sharp decline in intelligence test scores in the course of a longitudinal study tend to be those persons who will die within the next five years. It should come as no surprise that this hypothesis, carrying as it does a prophecy of doom that could set people into a needless frenzy if it proved wrong, has been subject to intense scrutiny from experimental psychologists since it was first proposed more than three decades ago. The consensus: the beguilingly simple theory is essentially correct. Many studies not only have confirmed the terminal drop hypothesis, but have refined it to such a point that some scientists have designated what they call a "critical loss" in certain measures of intelligence, a loss beyond which few individuals survive for more than five years.

The phrase "terminal drop" was coined in 1961 by gerontologist Robert Kleemeier, based on his observations of 13 elderly men. Kleemeier tested his subjects every two or three years for twelve years. Four of them died shortly after the study period was over; they proved, in retrospect, to have been those with the greatest and most rapid declines in cognitive ability. Kleemeier attributed this decline to a "terminal drop" that presaged death. The most elaborate confirmation of this initial work came from Germany, where the husband-and-wife team of Klaus and Ruth Riegel studied 380 men and women living near Hamburg. The subjects were tested in 1956, 1961, and 1966. By the time of the second testing, 62 subjects had died. Of the survivors, only 102 returned for a second testing in 1961, and those whose scores had dropped the most since the 1956 session were most likely to die within the next five years. Further, of the 116 original participants who were alive in 1961 but refused to return for further testing, 43 percent were dead by 1966—compared with just 25 percent of those subjects who returned for the 1961 tests. The Riegels theorized that many of the 116 resisters had already begun their terminal drop, and were aware that they would perform poorly if they submitted to a new round of intelligence tests.

Lissy Jarvik and her co-workers found that a generalized terminal drop in intelligence is less predictive of death than is a "critical loss" in only a few essential skills. They defined critical loss as a decline in two of the following three measures of intelligence: an annual decrement of 10 percent or more on the Wechsler-Bellevue subtest on similarities; an annual decrement of 2 percent or more on the Wechsler-Bellevue subtest on digit symbol substitution; and any decline at all on the Stanford-Binet subtest of vocabulary.

The critical loss measure proved its predictive value when Jarvik used it to assess which twins in a group of 26 twin pairs would die first. The twins had participated in a large-scale longitudinal study, so Jarvik could determine those individuals in whom a critical loss had appeared over time. Of the 30 twins (15 pairs) in whom Jarvik observed no critical loss in 1971, 27 were alive five years later. Of the 22 (11 pairs) in which one twin had manifested a critical loss, 10 twins from 10 different pairs were dead within five years—in each case, the twin who had already demonstrated intellectual decline.

Why does the terminal drop occur? Some scientists theorize that the physical illnesses at work that will soon kill the individual have an impact, too, on the cognitive capacities of the brain. Others say that intelligence changes are not merely a by-product of some other primary decline, but are an integral part of the processes preceding death.

At least one psychologist, M. A. Lieberman, assigns blame neither to a changing body nor to a changing brain but to a changing personality that also evolves in one's final years. Lieberman administered personality tests every three or four weeks to the residents of a home for the aged in Chicago. He compared the scores of those who died within three months of completing five test sessions with the scores of those still alive at least one year after completing ten test sessions. "Individuals approaching death pull away from those around them," he discovered, because they are "preoccupied in an attempt to hold themselves together—to reduce the experience of chaos." The non-survivors, said Lieberman, had lost their ability to cope with complex environments.

The most important factor in predicting death, he found, was not the absolute ability of an individual to cope with stress, but the loss of a previously demonstrated ability over time. This throws into relief the questions to be asked in the next two chapters. When an individual loses the skills, personality, and intelligence he or she once had, how does one determine whether the losses are due to illness, "senility," or simply old age? The distinction is a crucial one, because a mistaken assumption that any loss is inevitable with age, or is due to the irreversible condition called "senility," can lead to tragedy.

⋆ *4* ⋆

Pseudosenility

Like 1.3 million other old men and women, Mr. G. lives in a nursing home. Like more than half of them, he is classified as having Alzheimer's disease. He spends his days as he spends his nights: in a small, semi-private room, staring at the ceiling, staying in bed unless a nurse or orderly comes by to sit him up and strap him in a chair. His roommate is a ranter; he howls at the world, and when he wets his bed, he cries. Mr. G. is better off. He at least can feed himself. But his dentures haven't fit him right since his spell in the hospital four years back, so he drools a lot. When Mr. G.'s son and daughter-in-law come to visit, which is seldom, Mr. G. tends to forget his daughter-in-law's name, forgets why they've come, forgets why he's there.

The tragedy of Mr. G.'s story is not that he, like so many other elderly persons, has lost his ability to think. The tragedy is that his decline need not have happened. Because Mr. G. — a composite of at least 300,000 old people in nursing homes today — is suffering from senile symptoms that are the result of a physical disease in another part of his body, a disease that is probably 100 percent reversible.

As recently as five years ago, the most common diagnosis for an old man or woman like Mr. G. was a non-diagnosis — "senility." But today, a fancier sounding phrase is replacing that term, as more and more doctors and patients come to realize that, as a medical condition, "senility" simply does not exist. In the 1980s, a patient like Mr. G. is apt to receive a diagnosis that sounds like a true diagnosis but that is probably being bandied about far too freely — the diagnosis of Alzheimer's disease .

Alzheimer's disease is in danger of becoming "the new senility," a handy wastebasket category into which frustrated doctors can dump all the confused elderly patients who perplex them. What we have here is a variation of the old adage, "Give a man a hammer, and every problem begins to look like a nail." The physician's new, handy hammer is Alzheimer's disease, a diagnosis the public readily understands and accepts as scientific enough. But Alzheimer's disease is a diagnosis of doom. Physicians must resist making it until all other possibilities have been eliminated.

If the underlying cause of so-called senility is detected in time, hundreds of thousands of the people we now glibly diagnose as Alzheimer's patients could be restored to healthy mental functioning. A wide range of physical illnesses, all treatable, may cause confusion, disorientation, and memory loss in the aged. The illness could be as simple to treat as a hormonal imbalance or an infection, or it could require surgery, as does hydrocephalus ("water on the brain"). As many as 100 reversible physical conditions affect the aged brain even before they affect the target organ, says geriatrician Richard Besdine of the Harvard Medical School. But physicians, trained in the textbook diagnostic skills that link cause and effect for the "average" adult, often miss the true cause of the senile symptoms. Many doctors think a cause is hardly worth looking for. To them, confusion in an elderly patient is much like suicide in Philadelphia was to the comedian W. C. Fields: redundant.

But textbook diagnostic skills will not suffice in treating the elderly, who defy the "classic case." Sudden confusion in an old man or woman could mask just about any disorder—and that's where the medical art of "differential diagnosis," choosing the most likely diagnosis from among several probable ones, must come into play. "Elderly brains are very vulnerable to insults elsewhere in the body," says Besdine. "Diseases in the young and middle-aged may be straightforward; in the elderly, the brain might show the first signs of illness."

Sometimes the illnesses that seemed most simple to detect when they were taught in medical school become chameleons in the aged patient. According to the textbooks, when a fifty-year-old has a heart attack, chest pain is quick and direct. But 15 percent of elderly heart attack victims, says Besdine, show no sign other than confusion.

Similarly, hypoglycemia—low blood sugar that can lead to diabetic coma—usually causes weakness, dizziness, cold clammy sweats, and rapid heartbeat in the young and middle-aged. In the elderly, however, the only symptom may again be confusion. Infections can exist in the elderly without fever or an elevated white-blood-cell count. Hyperthyroidism may be present without the characteristic overactivity and protruding eyes found in young hyperthyroid patients. Appendicitis may occur without pain. Malnutrition, anemia, renal failure, vitamin deficiency—diseases affecting every part of the body can mimic senility in the elderly.

Sometimes complicated, expensive, and even risky procedures and tests are necessary before a conscientious doctor can with confidence rule out all explanations for senile symptoms except the final one—senile dementia. But many doctors fail to order all the right measurements and lab tests. Some even fail to look for the obvious causes of confusion, such as overmedication. In all likelihood, these physicians aren't especially sloppy, or lazy, or insensitive to their patients' distress or the distress of their patients' families. They're just ignorant about the long list of possible causes of confusion in the elderly. So the doctors are quick to call their old, confused patients senile, using a term that means nothing more than "old," as though it were a diagnosis.

"It's unforgivable," says Besdine. "Senility is not a diagnosis, it's a description. How many middle-aged men, if they went to a doctor complaining of chest pain, would be satisfied with a diagnosis of 'substernal distress of early middle years'?" And, one might add, how many doctors would offer such a diagnosis? But the standards applied to the aged are often different from those applied to everyone else—and doctors as well as relatives of the elderly are all too quick to make tragic decisions that can sentence patients like Mr. G. to a lifetime of needless emptiness.

Sloppy treatment of the aged derives from negative attitudes toward aging. Medical schools are prime breeding grounds for such attitudes. Quick cures and dramatic recoveries are pursued at most teaching hospitals, and the slow-to-mend elderly are cast off as unrewarding and uninteresting. Surveys show that the attitudes of medical students toward the elderly deteriorate markedly in medical school—a particularly poignant comment on a generation of doctors who can expect at least 40 percent of their patients to be over sixty-five.

As we shall see in chapter 8, some medical students have pushed for change in their curricula in recent years, and courses in geriatrics are among the most popular new electives offered. But medical schools on the whole are slow to change. Of 126 medical schools in the country, only two had an endowed professorship in geriatrics by the beginning of the 1980s, and just 85 or so had courses specifically in geriatrics, which were almost all electives. "Medical schools are still Peter Pan–like," says Robert N. Butler, chairman of the nation's first — and, to date, only — separate department of geriatrics, at the Mount Sinai Medical Center in New York. "They still deny the realities of aging in America."

Until the medical schools change, doctors will remain the wholesale purveyors of a condition that one gerontologist has dubbed "pseudosenility." They will remain ignorant about the treatable diseases that might account for the agitation of the eighty-six-year-old woman in the office waiting room or the disorientation of the seventy-two-year-old man on the hospital ward. They will persist in tossing all such unappealing, apparently uncooperative and incurable patients into the meaningless nondiagnostic heap of "senility."

Senility: The Great Imitator

Dozens of treatable illnesses cause confusion in the aged. How, then, is one to know whether senile symptoms are due to a reversible disease, to a serious but untreatable condition, or simply to the ravages of the years? The best clue is timing. The more rapid the onset of symptoms, the more likely it is that they are due to a reversible disease. If Mother "suddenly is not herself"; if Uncle Henry begins acting "senile" a few days after his prostate operation; if Grandma, who lives alone and rarely gets out, seems not to recognize her grandson on his quarterly visit, even though she was fine three months before—then these people are not necessarily just getting old. There may be a distinct problem—be it a vitamin deficiency or a blood clot on the brain—that can account for the apparently unaccountable.

In the art of differential diagnosis, the first thing doctors do is test for the most likely explanation for a particular set of symptoms. This way, the odds are on the side of finding a definitive answer. Doctors try, too, to test for treatable illnesses first, hoping against hope that the condition can at least be reversed. In the case of an old person who suddenly becomes confused, three probable diagnoses fit the conditions of being both common and reversible: drug toxicity, endocrine or metabolic disorders, and depression. Only after these common findings have been investigated and eliminated should a physician begin looking for the more exotic explanations.

Drug Toxicity: Iatrogenic Senility

"Doctors pour drugs of which they know little, to cure diseases of which they know less, into human beings of whom they know nothing." Voltaire's aphorism is especially true of physicians treating the elderly today, as the statistics of misdiagnosis and misprescription attest. The older you are, the more hazardous is a contact with the medical profession. The physician's inside joke that "a hospital is no place for sick people" is no joke for the aged: One study of 500 hospitalized elderly patients found that 146 of them (29.2 percent) experienced "untoward reactions" to hospitalization, and 28 percent of those reactions were directly attributable to drugs.

At the Johns Hopkins University Hospital adverse drug reactions were identified in 11.8 percent of the middle-aged patients (aged forty-one to fifty), but in fully 24 percent of the patients over eighty. In a larger study of 1,160 patients at a Belfast hospital, the findings were similar: 10.2 percent of patients of all ages were found to encounter adverse drug reactions, but once again the proportion increased with age, to 15.4 percent for patients over sixty, and 20.3 percent for those over seventy.

"In my experience, iatrogenic—doctor-induced—confusional states do happen, and they happen quite frequently," says Thomas Kalchthaler, medical director of the St. Joseph's Nursing Home in Yonkers, New York. Kalchthaler has developed this rule for the elderly patients he treats: "Whenever a new patient shows up here in a confusional state, the first thing I do is check the medications."

Often, stopping all or most medications is the first step back to full mental functioning for the aged. This is especially true of the psychotherapeutic drugs—drugs that, ironically, may have been prescribed to treat the very symptoms they later created. A study conducted by B. M. Learoyd at an Australian psychogeriatric unit found that of 236 elderly patients admitted, 16 percent were suffering the direct effects of psychoactive drugs. Seven patients were confused or excessively sedated; 14 experienced agitation, paranoia, and aggression; and 16 had psychic disturbances along with such physical symptoms as respiratory depression, urinary retention, and intestinal obstruction. According to Learoyd, each patient improved enough to be discharged from the hospital when the offending medication was significantly reduced or stopped completely.

Why are the elderly so exquisitely sensitive to adverse drug effects? For one thing, they take more medications than young people, so the odds are they will encounter more difficulty. Second, they tend not to follow doctor's instructions when taking their medicine, often because they never understood the instructions in the first place. Third, the doctor's instructions themselves are often wrong, since many physicians fail to account for age-related changes in drug metabolism and excretion and may set dosages at levels that are nearly toxic for the elderly. And last, even if the patient follows his doctor's instructions to the letter, and even if the doctor keeps the prescribed dosages sufficiently low, the older patient is statistically more likely than the younger patient to encounter the problem of drug interactions—a complex and often debilitating event (which occurs as well in younger people) resulting from the pharmacologic interplay of different medications in the body.

We will consider each reason in turn, bearing in mind this fact: When an adverse drug reaction does occur in the elderly, it usually turns up as a change in mental function. Certain common drugs, such as digitalis, diuretics, oral anti-diabetes drugs, analgesics, steroids, and sedatives, actually induce organic brain disorders which, if not corrected in time, could lead to irreparable damage. Other drugs may simply throw off the physiological balance just enough to tip the most precarious element—mental functioning. Finally, some drugs may create physical side effects (usually an increased slowing of response, which further exaggerates the normal slowing down of age) that are distressing enough to confuse and disorient an elderly person who hasn't been sufficiently warned to expect these reactions.

The elderly are by far the largest group of drug consumers. The National Health Care Expenditure Study reported in

1982 that each person over sixty-five who was on medication spent an average of $93 a year on prescription drugs and refills—compared to $46 per person per year for the population as a whole. That year, when the elderly made up about 12 percent of the U.S. population, they paid for 25 percent of all drugs and drug sundries. In Great Britain, a similar pattern exists. In 1976, when the elderly were 12 percent of the population, they accounted for some 30 percent of the national expenditure for prescription drugs.

With the bulk of medications being sold to the elderly it's no wonder that physicians estimate that persons over sixty-five run a twofold greater risk of adverse drug reactions than do younger patients. That risk is heightened by the drug-taking habits of the aged. Although the incidence of "noncompliance" (a physician-derived term, meaning failure to take medications exactly as instructed) is thought to be no higher among the elderly than among any other age group, it is still surprisingly high. And the effects can be more profound in old people who are already vulnerable, weak, and often experiencing several underlying chronic illnesses in addition to the one for which they're being medicated.

Researchers at two outpatient clinics, one in New York City and one in Seattle, found that a majority of elderly patients did in fact make mistakes in taking their prescribed medication and that those who did make mistakes usually made more than one at a time. At the general medical clinic of New York Hospital, D. Schwartz found that 59 percent of the patients over age sixty made an average of 2.6 medication errors each. Among these "noncompliant" patients, 26 percent made mistakes that were potentially quite serious. According to Schwartz, the most common mistake was failure to take the prescribed drug at all.

D. M. Parkin, a British physician, reported that of 130 elderly patients studied, 66 made errors in drug-taking ten days after leaving the hospital. The greatest problem, Parkin found, was lack of a clear understanding of the proper schedule, which occurred more than twice as often as simple failure to follow instructions.

Like patients in other age groups, the elderly fail to take medicine correctly for a variety of reasons. As Parkin emphasized, they may not understand doctor's orders—a problem aggravated by the cultural, educational, and language barriers that often exist between old people and their physicians. They may forget whether they took their pill from one morning to the next afternoon—a problem exacerbated by the awkward combination of growing forgetfulness with age, loss of routine to provide clues for memory, and the confusing array of pills and potions many older people must take. They may not have the money, or the energy, or the means of transportation, to keep a full supply of medications on hand, which could lead to deliberate skipping of pills in order to make the medicine last longer. Or they may not believe that the drug will make any difference in the way they feel—a belief confirmed by certain drugs, such as many anti-hypertension medications, that actually create more symptoms than they alleviate.

But even for those elderly people who follow doctor's orders conscientiously—employing, as many of these "compliant" patients do, such memory aids as tear-off calendars, notes, and individualized vials arranged by the day instead of by the drug—the orders themselves may be wrong. A surprising number of physicians still fail to understand that age-related changes in the body mean that drugs are utilized differently by older people, and may remain in the system for as much as 50 percent longer than in the "typical" adult for whom most recommended doses are set. For certain medications, a normal dose for a forty-year-old is an overdose for an eighty-year-old—and many doctors fail to make the proper adjustments when writing prescriptions. This is the cause of iatrogenic illness, and this is why the doctors themselves may at times be hazardous to health.

Most drugs are metabolized in the liver, bound to proteins in the cells and blood, distributed to body water or to muscles and bone (called lean body mass), and excreted through the kidney. At every step in this process, age-related changes in organ function and body distribution come into play. Total body water has been shown to decrease by 10 to 15 percent with age, while the amount of total body fat increases by 10 to 20 percent. "Alterations in body fat," says one geriatric pharmacologist, "might result in accumulation and prolongation of highly lipid-soluble drugs." Similarly, the level of albumin—a major protein present in virtually every cell—is 20 percent lower in the elderly, so the action of drugs such as meperidine and warfarin, which bind to cell protein on their way out of the body, is significantly prolonged. All these physiological changes alter the picture of drug distribution and elimination, since more of the medication remains circulating in the bloodstream for a longer period of time.

Liver function tends to remain intact throughout life, but the organ has been shown to become relatively smaller, and with a decreased blood flow, with age. In a classic study by Sheila Sherlock and her colleagues at the Postgraduate Medical School of London, liver blood flow was found to decrease by 1.5 percent a year throughout life, meaning that a sixty-five-year-old has 40 to 45 percent less blood flowing to his liver than does a twenty-five-year-old. Thus, drugs such as Valium (diazepam) that are metabolized through the liver may exhibit profound differences in the rate at which they are eliminated from body. Robert Vestal of the Boise (Idaho) Veterans Administration Hospital, an expert on drug metabolism in the aged, has compiled results of a series of experiments involving twenty-five drugs metabolized through the liver. Age-related changes were observed along two dimensions: biological half-life (the time it takes for one-half of the drug to be excreted from the body) and clearance (the rate at which the drug is totally eliminated). As seen in the following table, eleven of the drugs showed age-related differences in drug half-life in at least one of the studies Vestal surveyed, and nine showed differences in the rates of clearance.

Change in drug metabolism by an old liver is documented, Vestal says, by studies of the pain-killer antipyrine, a "model compound" for tests of this sort because its half-life and clearance rate are almost wholly dependent on liver metabolism. Several studies confirm a significantly prolonged half-life and reduced clearance rate for antipyrine with age. Vestal qualifies these findings, though, by pointing out that certain lifestyle changes that tend to accompany age—particularly reduced use of alcohol, caffeine, and cigarettes—may account for most of the observed changes.

At the Gerontology Research Center in Baltimore, researchers studied the function of another organ—the kidney. Here, even more dramatic changes with age were observed. In a typical ninety-year-old, the scientists found, the glomerular filtration rate (GFR), a measurement of the drug-clearing capacity of the kidney, is 35 percent lower than the GFR of a typical twenty-year-old, and may be reduced by as much as 50 percent. Because kidney function is so easily measured, Vestal suggests that physicians test all elderly patients' GFR before setting a dosage regimen for kidney-excreted medications such as penicillin, streptomycin, tetracycline, digoxin, practolol, sulfamethizole, and phenobarbital.

Unfortunately, there's no magic formula for prescribing drugs for the elderly, except the obvious: Be careful, start

ELIMINATION OF DRUGS VIA THE LIVER IN YOUNG AND OLD SUBJECTS

AGE-RELATED DIFFERENCES IN BIOLOGICAL HALF-LIFE

DIFFERENCES FOUND	NO DIFFERENCES FOUND
Acetaminophen	Imipramine
Acetanilid	Indomethacin
Aminopyrine	Isoniazid
Antipyrine	Lorazepam
Chlordiazepoxide	Morphine
Chlormethiazole	Nitrazepam
Desipramine	Oxasepam
Diazepam	Phenylbutazone
Lidocaine	Phenytoin
Lorazepam	Tolbutamide
Quinidine	Warfarin

AGE-RELATED DIFFERENCES IN TOTAL METABOLIC CLEARANCE

DIFFERENCES FOUND	NO DIFFERENCES FOUND
Acetaminophen	Acetaminophen
Antipyrine	Diazepam
Chlordiazepoxide	Ethanol
Chlormethiazole	Lidocaine
Phenylbutazone	Phenytoin
Phenytoin	Warfarin
Propranolol	
Quinidine	
Tolbutamide	

From Robert E. Vestal, "Aging and pharmacokinetics: Impact of altered physiology in the elderly," in *Physiology and Cell Biology of Aging*, A. Cherkin et al. (eds.), New York: Raven Press, 1979.

with the lowest possible dose, and, if you can, do away with certain medications altogether. "If a drug causes more symptoms than it alleviates," Vestal advises, "then it should not be used." Also, he urges his colleagues, "Strive for a diagnosis prior to treatment . . . [since] if the patient's symptoms are due to malnutrition, ill-fitting dentures, social deprivation, inability to pay for previously ordered medications, abuse or misuse of medications, additional drug therapy is only likely to complicate the situation." One would hope his advice were self-evident to doctors treating the elderly today, but, sadly, it is not. As Alexander Leaf, chief of medicine at the prestigious Massachusetts General Hospital has observed, "Even in our hospital, the number of elderly patients who suffer reactions to drugs administered while in the hospital is frightening." Many physicians simply do not know how to prescribe for the elderly.

In fairness to doctors, it must be said that old people present an additional wrinkle to the therapeutic plan—their tendency to be not simply sick, but sick with a variety of illnesses. "Multiple diseases are the rule rather than the exception in the elderly patient," Vestal says. "Superimposed upon old injuries, prior illness and past operations may be a variety of chronic disorders, such as cataracts, pernicious anemia, osteoarthritis, osteoporosis, atherosclerosis, and diabetes." More than 85 percent of Americans over age sixty-five are thought to suffer from one or more chronic conditions. A 1984 study of the National Center for Health Statistics found that chronic conditions led to a serious limitation of activity in nearly 40 percent of Americans over age sixty-five.

Because they suffer from multiple diseases, the elderly are multi-medicated. According to the Department of Health and Human Services, persons over age sixty-five take an average of 7.5 drugs *each*. "And as the number of medications taken increases," says Kalchthaler of St. Joseph's, "the chance of adverse drug reactions increases exponentially." This phenomenon is what physicians call drug-drug interaction, a confounding process that pharmacologists are just beginning to unravel. When it affects younger patients, its existence seems obvious; when it affects the elderly, it can, once again, produce symptoms that look like senility.

Consider this description from the *New England Journal of Medicine* of two middle-aged men referred to psychiatrist William E. Thornton with symptoms that looked very much like "senility":

> *[The first patient showed] symptoms of psychomotor retardation, inability to do arithmetic calculations, recent memory impairment, and ideas of reference with accompanying inappropriate suspiciousness. . . . [The second revealed] marked slowing of both motor and mental performance, transient disorientation to place and time, inability to concentrate, and intermittent ability to recognize his own handwriting.*

Because these patients were, respectively, a forty-three-year-old accountant and a forty-eight-year-old lawyer, Thornton was alerted by these symptoms and took a careful medical history. He found that each man had been taking methyldopa for years to treat hypertension, and that the symptoms began within a week of administration of haloperidol, a popular tranquilizer. Thornton stopped the haloperidol, and within seventy-two hours the symptoms cleared, and never returned.

If these two men had been in their seventies or eighties, the symptoms produced by this drug-drug interaction probably would have seemed unremarkable. It's unlikely they would even have been referred to Thornton for psychiatric care, much less have been deemed of sufficient interest to make the pages of a leading medical journal. But adverse

97

interactions of this sort are far more likely to occur in the aged than in the middle-aged. As Vestal observes, "It is not unusual for a patient to receive two or more drugs of the same type or with similar side effects—perhaps prescribed by the same or different clinicians. For example, antidepressants, antipsychotic agents, antihistamines, and nonprescription 'cold' remedies and sedative preparations all have anticholinergic properties [blocking the flow of information in the brain, which could inhibit such disparate functions as tear and saliva production, muscle tone, and secretions of hormones]. Their effects may be additive."

Endocrine Disorders: Regulators Gone Awry

The line blurs between iatrogenic senility—mental decline caused by drugs that doctors prescribe—and the next most prevalent cause of reversible dementia: endocrine and metabolic disorder. The body's endocrine glands—the thyroid, parathyroids, pancreas, adrenal glands, pituitary, ovaries, and testes—are responsible for keeping the body in a state of equanimity called homeostasis. Old age itself usually interrupts this delicate balance between gland function and hormone secretion, but another frequent cause of endocrine disturbance is medication.

Ironically, one of the most common causes of hypothyroidism—underfunctioning of the thyroid gland, which produces a senility-like syndrome in persons of all ages—is Iodine 131, a medication once used in the treatment of the very disorder it now seems to induce. Richard Mahler, an endocrinologist at the Eisenhower Medical Center in California, says that hypothyroidism is becoming more and more prevalent in his elderly patients, who come to him with "lethargy, somnolence, and forgetfulness . . . all often easily assumed to be part of the aging process." Mahler's theory is that many of these patients were treated for hypothyroidism in the 1950s with Iodine 131, which has been shown to cause thyroid dysfunction about seventeen years after treatment in as many as half the patients exposed to it.

Another explanation for the increasing prevalence of hypothyroidism in the aged, Mahler says, is the popularity of the antidepressive drug lithium. Lithium has been shown to interfere not only with the function of the thyroid gland, but also with the regulation of glucose metabolism. It can induce a diabetes-like problem called diabetes insipidus. This disease, like hypothyroidism, produces a set of mental symptoms that look like senility in patients of any age—and are often diagnosed as senility in those patients unlucky enough to be chronologically old.

The symptoms of these disorders are striking, and to the uninitiated they are dead ringers for "senile dementia." Consider this old woman, described in *Geriatrics* magazine by two Boston University physicians:

> One very warm June day in upstate New York, a public health nurse arrived to aid in the disposition of an elderly woman who had come to the attention of the Health Department because of an odor emanating from her apartment. As soon as the door was opened a blast of hot air escaped from the room. The woman was found lying in bed under a number of blankets complaining of the cold. This elderly lady was thought to be just "senile" by a series of health care professionals before one physician asked for a determination of her thyroid status. The result of the test confirmed the diagnosis of profound hypothyroidism, a very treatable disease.

The clue to her endocrine disorder had been her internal body thermostat, which obviously was malfunctioning in a bizarre way. But because she was old, most doctors, nurses, and mental health workers with whom she came in contact simply assumed she was a batty old lady who liked to complain.

For some reason, hyperthyroidism, in which the gland secretes *too much* thyroid hormone, looks very much like hypothyroidism in elderly patients. In the middle-aged, the classic case of hyperthyroidism is a jittery, easily irritated, agitated individual with protruding eyes (called exophthalmos) and warm, moist skin. Everything moves too fast: the patient loses weight despite a voracious appetite, tires easily despite an incessant need for activity, has a rapid heartbeat and high blood pressure. The classic middle-aged hypothyroid individual, in contrast, works in slow motion, experiencing listlessness, slow speech, weakness. In hypothyroidism, the skin is usually dry, and the patient is extraordinarily sensitive to heat and cold because the body cannot adapt to outside stimuli quickly enough.

But in the elderly, these classic descriptions are worthless. Old people tend to exhibit what physicians call "apathetic hyperthyroidism"—in other words, a decrease rather than an increase in nervous energy. The characteristic exophthalmos is almost always missing from elderly hyperthyroid patients. In fact, old people who suffer from any derangement of thyroid function, either too much or too little, have only one symptom that occurs frequently enough to be called typical: the changes in mental function that look like symptoms of senility.

In a classic study of hyperthyroid and hypothyroid patients conducted by researchers at the University of North Carolina, the picture that emerged for many of the patients was that of a typical senile person. Most of the seventeen individuals in the study were middle-aged, and their symptoms of loss of recent memory, inability to concentrate sufficiently to do simple arithmetic, depression, anxiety, and confusion were unexpected enough to raise physicians' concerns. Like Thornton's two middle-aged patients, the North Carolina patients were by and large spared a casual non-diagnosis of "senility" because they had the good fortune to be in their forties and fifties. But if they had been twenty or thirty years older, they might not have even made it to the clinic for treatment.

According to Mahler, several other endocrine disorders may also look like senility to the uninformed.

> *I recall seeing a 73-year-old patient some years ago in New York, who had been taken to a nursing home because every morning, on awakening, she became confused, disoriented, somewhat belligerent, and exceedingly uncooperative. This caused her family great difficulty in dealing with her. It was assumed that more than likely she was not salvageable, and the family placed her into a nursing home. It was only with routine blood testing that her fasting blood sugar was observed to be below 40 milligrams [a normal fasting blood sugar is in the range of about 100 milligrams]. On further evaluation she proved to have a functioning islet cell adenoma [a benign tumor of the pancreas] with documented hyperinsulinism [oversecretion of insulin by the pancreas, resulting in dangerously low levels of blood sugar after a long period without food—such as eight hours of sleep]. Unusual, yes, but a point certainly worth keeping in mind.*

Similarly, if the adrenal gland malfunctions, due either to normal aging or to the effects of drugs or coexisting disease, the resulting glucose deficiency may cause behavior that looks like senility. And hyperparathyroidism—overactivity of the parathyroid gland in the base of the brain, which stimulates secretion of the sex hormones—causes an excess of calcium to circulate in the body, which in turn may also produce senility-like symptoms.

101

Depression: The Common Cold of Mental Illness

Depression is the most prevalent mental disorder in the United States. An estimated 15 percent of the population will suffer at least one episode that requires medical intervention. Depression also is a psychiatric chameleon. Any number of psychological or physical complaints may be due to depression, ranging from insomnia, lethargy, and loss of self-esteem to headaches, abdominal pain, urinary problems, and chest constriction.

What makes depression particularly poignant is that it lends added power to social stereotypes of how people behave. As we saw in chapter 3, depressed teenagers have been shown to engage in activity characteristic of the typical "juvenile delinquent"—rebelliousness, restlessness, rowdiness. Depressed older people have been shown to complain of mental changes that are part of the senility stereotype, particularly complaints of memory loss. "These people have a pervasive sense of no-goodness," says Ernest Gruenberg, a psychiatrist at Johns Hopkins University. So, lacking faith in their own ideas about how to behave, depressed people turn to an available stereotype as a reference point for self-description. In the aged, Gruenberg says, "that sense of no-goodness comes out when they say, 'I can't remember. I don't know. I'm senile.' "

It's easy to see why old people would be depressed. Suddenly stripped of roles, prestige, power, and self-esteem, the aged must deal with an ongoing sense of loss. Their grief is progressive as they mourn lost spouses, friends, relatives—and their own lost youth. The prevalence of depression in the elderly—and the importance of the disorder as a matter of life and death—is evident in the suicide statistics in the United States. Persons over sixty-five, who are 12 percent of the population, today commit 25 percent of the successful suicides. Old men, whose fall from grace after forced retirement is most dramatic, show an especially striking pattern of suicide. The suicide rate for white men in 1982, when the overall rate for all ages was 12.3 per 100,000, was 31 per 100,000 men between sixty-five and seventy-four, 45 per 100,000 men between seventy-five and eighty-four, and 50 per 100,000 men over eighty-five.

But some physicians who have been alerted to the fact that senile symptoms may, in the aged, mask an underlying depression are in danger of turning depression into a new "wastebasket diagnosis" for the elderly. Rather than exhausting all possible medical conditions before making a diagnosis, some doctors are assuming that confusion, forgetfulness, and disorientation probably mean an old person is depressed—and that depression is a reasonable, inherent reaction to old age. This attitude is nearly as damaging as is the assumption that "senility," and its attendant mental changes, is part and parcel of old age. Indeed, in some sense it might be more damaging, because with it comes the cavalier use of antidepressant drugs for the elderly, drugs that in some aged patients can lead to distressing side effects.

"It is a mistake to assume that depressions in late life are caused by unhappy environmental circumstances, or just being old," says Raymond Adams, chief of neurology at Harvard's Massachusetts General Hospital. This belief leads to a kind of fatalism that the aged do not deserve. "As a working principle," Adams says, "a persistent anxious depression should never be regarded as a reaction to environment, but rather as a disease state." When old people begin to lose ability to function, to maintain previous jobs or activities, to relate to family and friends, Adams says the physician must assume that the patient "probably has a disease, and deserves to be studied in a hospital where there are physicians competent in the diagnosis of the nervous system. No longer is it sufficient to let these people be passed off as nervous and sent for treatment by psychotherapists. All of these patients should be studied medically."

If medical examination reveals no physical problem, many doctors then believe they "owe" their older patients a trial of antidepressant medication. The crucial step here is the prior elimination of all possible medical disease. Certain mood-elevating drugs sometimes help lift a depression in the older patient, though, as we have seen, old people are especially sensitive to the adverse side effects of psychoactive medications. Other techniques used to treat psychological problems in younger patients also work well for the old, including psychotherapy, psychoanalysis, group psychotherapy, behavioral modification, physical and occupational therapy, family counseling, and sex counseling.

For some old people, depression is the result of sheer, overwhelming loneliness, and a prolonged visit with the physician may be sufficient to ease it. For others, more intensive therapy is called for—and, contrary to the beliefs of many mental health professionals, such therapy is useful no matter how old the patient is.

The psychiatric profession is notorious for its collective attitude that aged, depressed patients aren't worth the therapeutic investment. Psychiatrist Robert Butler of Mount Sinai Medical Center in New York is ruthless in his condemnation of his peers' treatment of the elderly:

> They are so often impatient and irritable with their older patients for not responding swiftly to their ministrations. It would not occur to them to push for such rapid improvement in younger patients. In part, they fear the implacable clock; there will not be enough time in which to work. In part, they reflect the notion that old people cannot change. Ironically,

part of the reason old people are eminently capable of change is that they stand so near to death. They have things to accomplish before it is too late.

The psychiatric profession has changed somewhat in recent years (Butler made that statement in 1975). Evidence of the new interest in the elderly is the overnight growth of a section on geropsychiatry, first formed at the 1979 meeting of the American Psychiatric Association (APA). The section was announced at the first plenary session of the APA meeting, and within two days, 400 psychiatrists had joined.

One still-controversial issue in the treatment of depression in the elderly is the appropriateness of electroshock therapy. Some psychiatrists, such as Ernest Gruenberg of Johns Hopkins, advocate shock treatment if all else fails. "You must be more careful with electroshock therapy for the elderly, just as you must be more careful with surgery," Gruenberg says. "But it's wrong to think, 'Oh, no, never electric shock,' just because the patient's old."

Geriatricians emphasize that an old man's or old woman's psychological profile is usually a reiteration of his or her lifelong personality; as one psychiatrist put it, old people are "exactly what they were all their lives; if they were rats, they become worse rats." But depression in the elderly cannot be explained as an individual personality quirk, a culmination of a lifetime of insecurity and moroseness. The suicide statistics and the prevalence of depressive disorders in the aged bespeak a larger, society-based cause for the emotional breakdown of age. If depression in the elderly is to be prevented, the place of the old in Western society will have to be reassigned. People tossed to the bottom of the heap, particularly people who had once shared the limelight with the rest of us, at present have little recourse but withdrawal and despair.

Other Reversible Causes of Pseudosenility

Mrs. T. probably will never know how close she came to becoming just another tragic statistic.

> *"She was a 75-year-old woman who looked like a paranoid schizophrenic," recalls her psychiatrist, Robert Kahn. "In fact, another psychiatrist here was convinced she was a chronic, lifelong schizophrenic. But her family kept insisting that she had never had psychiatric symptoms before, so we checked her further. It turned out she had an acutely infected kidney. We treated her kidney, and her psychosis cleared up."*

For every 100 elderly patients who come to their doctors with the symptoms of senility—forgetfulness, confusion, disorientation, delirium, hallucinations—at least 10 of them, and perhaps as many as 30, are not senile. They are not psychotic. They are physically sick.

Once drug toxicity has been ruled out and the patient's hormone functioning has been checked, there are still dozens of reversible illnesses that could be causing the senile behavior. Kidney infection is one, as are other infections ranging from stomach flu to urinary tract infection to pneumonia to meningitis. Infections are particularly hard to detect in the elderly, since often they don't even produce a fever—just confusion.

Environmental pollutants such as carbon monoxide, lead, and mercury also can cause confusion and other behavioral changes in the aged. Vitamin deficiency, especially of vitamin B12 or folic acid, can produce pseudosenility, as can other results of malnutrition, a common condition among old people. They tend to live alone and eat alone, have limited incomes, encounter age-related changes in taste buds that make many foods taste bitter or sour, and often have trouble even getting to the market.

Anemia, a general term meaning a qualitative or quantitative blood deficiency, is another cause of pseudosenility. But it is a condition that is both difficult to define—how much blood is enough blood for an old person?—and difficult to diagnose. A wide range of disorders may cause anemia (which is, strictly speaking, a symptom, and not a diagnosis). Among them are malnutrition, blood vessel compression, blood clot, internal bleeding, and cancer. Symptoms of anemia are vague and may be absent in the aged; once more, old people may show no sign of the physical disorder other than confusion.

The very conditions that are most treatable in the aged—conditions such as gallstones, hepatitis, urinary retention, dehydration, fecal impaction—can, tragically, masquerade as the one condition most feared because it seems the most untreatable. It seems a cruel irony indeed that the dominant symptom of almost every physical disorder of old age—confusion—is the symptom that most terrifies the elderly and their loved ones. Perhaps the prevalence of confusion as a symptom of geriatric disease accounts in part for the widespread acceptance of the belief that confusion is inevitable with age.

Why does the brain seem to be the first organ to show signs of stress, not only psychological and emotional stress but biological stress as well? Physicians like Besdine would say it's because the brain is the most changed, the weakest link in the body's chain and thus the first to break in times of strain. Psychiatrists like Kahn would cast it in a more personality-oriented light. They call the confusion "decompensation," a psychological reaction to stress in a system already operating at the brink. The aged body, Kahn says, can function only because of the individual's ability to "compensate" for a series of minor physical changes. This delicate balance, held taut by the string of personality, is

107

toppled when any kind of stress—be it depression, infection, a new drug, or a new life situation—makes individuals lose their grip on the compensatory mechanism they have evolved to date.

Diagnosing Pseudosenility

Whatever accounts for the prevalence of confusion as a primary symptom of so many problems, the fact remains that families and doctors must be on the alert to look for a reason for an old person's senile behavior—a reason with more substance than the typical "Well, what do you expect at your age." To find it, physicians must embark upon what geriatricians Knight Steel and Robert Feldman call "a compulsively detailed physical examination."

Even the basic first steps, such as taking the patient's temperature, blood pressure, and pulse rate, could turn up subtle abnormalities which themselves could account for the confusion. Steel and Feldman suggest a complete roster of laboratory tests, including measures of liver and kidney function, chest X ray, electrocardiogram, stool guaiac test, serology, thyroid function test, and determinations of blood levels of calcium, phosphorus, sodium chloride, potassium, carbon dioxide, serum B12, and folate. In some cases, more costly tests such as electroencephalography (EEG), skull films, brain scans, and arteriography may also be warranted. Steel and Feldman recommend computerized tomography (CT)—in which X-ray slices of the brain are rearranged by a computer into a three-dimensional picture—for most elderly patients who are confused. The study is expensive—upwards of $500—but, as Steel and Feldman point out, "the cost of institutionalizing a patient for six or more years greatly exceeds that."

One thought must be prominent in the minds of physicians working on a diagnosis of confused elderly patients: a wrong diagnosis, too quick a decision on the side of inevitability, is not simply a mistake—it is a sentence of death. Delay in pinpointing the underlying cause of apparent "senility" can turn a reversible condition into a permanent one.

As gerontologists spread the word, one hopes that physicians will learn to be more scrupulous in the differential diagnosis of confusion in the elderly. "The elderly demand that we be much more professional in our treatment of them," observes psychiatrist Robert Kahn. "They're much more challenging, much less routine. And it's very, very important that we make these distinctions [between reversible and irreversible causes of confusion.] This is not just an intellectual game."

For every 100 confused old people who show up in the doctor's office, perhaps 10 or 20 or 30 of them can be treated and cured. But we must remember the reality of those other 70 to 90 patients, the ones who are in fact suffering a disease that will render them gradually unable to remember, think, reason, or care for themselves. Even though our treatment of the aged has created a good many senile symptoms, and even though our misdiagnosis has ignored a good many cases where those symptoms could be cured, there remains a sizable minority of the aged population who have all the symptoms we mean when we talk about "senility." These are the people with Alzheimer's disease.

❧ 5 ❧

Alzheimer's Disease: The Real Senile Dementia

The whimpering sounded as though it came from a child. But there were no children here at the St. Joseph's Nursing Home in Yonkers, New York—only old people finishing their lunch. They huddled in wheelchairs, slumped at tables, lay in stretchers that carried traces of soup and spit. They muttered, mouths sunk in wrinkles, and some hugged nurses and orderlies or dozed off in the corner. "Stay clear," warned one old man, a lunch tray across his lap. "Bad mood, bad mood."

The sunshine that bathed the room added a sad irony to the scene, a scene that fills many of our darkest nightmares. All the old people in this room have a disease called senile dementia.

The most common form of senile dementia, Alzheimer's disease, has become so well-known in the past few years that it is in danger of becoming what the word "senility" itself used to be—a wastebasket term that says nothing about the cause or treatment of particular symptoms. Our goal in this chapter is to describe the possible causes and treatments of Alzheimer's disease, a distressingly common condition whose incidence increases sharply with age. The longer we live, the greater our chances of developing Alzheimer's disease; perhaps as many as 20 percent of Americans who live past eighty will show brain changes and behavioral changes that can be traced to the disease. But the awful commonness of Alzheimer's disease must not let us lose sight of one important truth: Senile dementia is not the result of normal aging; it is a pathological process that most people never experience, no matter how long they live.

For the 3 million or more Americans who develop Alzheimer's disease, life can be hell—and it can be even more hellish for their families, who by and large care for their loved ones until the debilitation is more than they can bear. The process of the disease is inevitable, moving (sometimes slowly, sometimes quickly) from such apparently harmless traits as forgetfulness, slovenliness, and withdrawal, to the more profound changes of inability to reason, loss of judgment, loss of memory, loss of orientation, inability to calculate, and, finally, inability to care for oneself or even to remember one's own name. Frequently, the final stages of Alzheimer's are accompanied by incontinence (loss of control over bodily functions, either of the bladder or colon or both), and this last step, or its imminence, is often the one that leads to institutionalization of the patient.

Alzheimer's disease accounts for an estimated 60 percent of all cases of senile dementia. That leaves another 40 percent of old persons with dementia that cannot be traced to Alzheimer's disease. Roughly one-half of them are suffering from multi-infarct dementia, a vascular disorder that once was mislabeled "hardening of the arteries of the brain." In multi-infarct dementia, the brain suffers a series of little strokes that lead to loss of blood flow, and hence loss of function, in those regions where the strokes occur. This form of dementia is usually accompanied by vascular problems elsewhere in the body. Other dementias are, like Alzheimer's disease, diseases of the brain cells themselves. Scientists have clues about the origins of many of them: Korsakoff's psychosis, which has been traced to a lifetime of alcoholism; Huntington's disease, carried on a single gene as an autosomal dominant trait; dementia pugilistica, also known as the "punch-drunk syndrome," which occurs after the repeated head trauma of a boxing career: Creutzfeld-Jakob disease and kuru, each of which is probably caused by a slow-acting virus; and Parkinson's disease, caused by a deficiency of the neurotransmitter dopamine.

Like Alzheimer's disease, most of these dementias are progressive and incurable. Multi-infarct dementia occasionally responds to blood-thinning drugs, but as for the others, doctors can offer little in the way of therapy. They are making some strides in minimizing the accompanying problems of the disease, such as incontinence, but so far the basic brain degeneration cannot be stopped. Although claims of success with certain drugs and techniques, such as vitamin E, choline, Deanol, Piracetam, and hyperbaric oxygen chambers, have been made in recent years, these methods haven't yet stood up to rigorous scientific scrutiny. The best a doctor can prescribe today to the family is patience.

Tragically, victims of Alzheimer's disease sometimes house their sick minds in relatively healthy bodies. They can survive for ten years or more in a state of utterly dependent mental emptiness. In severe cases, though, the disease is a fast worker, generally reducing life expectancy by one-half; 95 percent of its victims over age seventy are dead within eight years of diagnosis.

The cause of Alzheimer's disease still eludes scientists. Although there has been much research interest recently, questions, not answers, have been raised so far. The family of one ex-butcher who died of Alzheimer's disease wonders whether his taste for calves' brains didn't make him ill; perhaps he ate a brain that had itself been diseased? The family of another man with Alzheimer's disease believes his bout with an extraordinary high fever of 106° F, which made him unconscious for three days when he was in his forties, caused some permanent brain damage that is now revealing itself as a progressive dementia. The families of all patients with Alzheimer's disease grope through the family tree looking for relatives who also died after undergoing strange mental changes: they wonder whether the disease is hereditary, and whether they and their children are at risk.

Experts can offer them little guidance in sifting the possible from the improbable. At this point, the families' guesses about the cause of Alzheimer's disease are almost as good as the doctors'.

Alzheimer's: A Leading Killer

The deadly powers of Alzheimer's disease are generally hidden to public health officials. As "cause of death" listed on the death certificate, Alzheimer's disease, like other chronic illnesses, appears rather infrequently—in 1977 just over 2,000 deaths out of nearly 2 million overall were attributed directly to Alzheimer's disease. But neurologist Robert Katzman, chairman of the Department of Neuroscience at the University of California at San Diego, estimates that Alzheimer's disease is the cause of 100,000 to 120,000 deaths a year in the United States. The illnesses listed as cause of death, he says—bronchitis, pneumonia, pulmonary edema—are only incidental players in the Alzheimer's disease patient's steady deterioration. If Katzman's figures are correct, that would make Alzheimer's disease the nation's fourth or fifth leading killer.

For all that Alzheimer's disease is such a powerful killer, however, most persons over sixty-five run a very small chance of developing the disorder—just about 5 percent of a random sampling of the elderly. The most clearly described risk factor is a history of Alzheimer's disease in a close family member. The closeness of the association depends on the closeness of the family relationship: among twins whose co-twins already have Alzheimer's disease, for example, identical twins run a higher risk of developing the disease themselves than do non-identical twins. One large-scale study conducted in Sweden concluded that a seventy-five-year-old with no history of Alzheimer's disease in the family runs a 1.2 percent chance of developing Alzheimer's, while a seventy-five-year-old whose sibling or parent had Alzheimer's runs a 5.7 percent chance. At the age of ninety, the likelihood of developing Alzheimer's disease increases to 5 percent for the general population, and 23 percent for a close relative of someone with Alzheimer's disease. This pattern of "familial clustering" need not mean there is a genetic component to Alzheimer's, though that now seems the most likely explanation. But it could also mean that something in the family's environment—exposure to the same disease-causing organisms, perhaps, or to the same environmental pollutants—could also be causing the clustering of the disease.

In the process of killing, Alzheimer's disease can, as geriatrician Robert Butler has put it, "rob the living of life itself." Without meaning to, patients with Alzheimer's disease demand the full time and attention of their families and other caretakers. "We put my mother to bed every evening," says one woman whose mother has Alzheimer's disease", and within a very short time—the record so far is twenty minutes later—she's back downstairs, dressed and ready to start the day. After we tell her it's still nighttime and manage to get her back to bed, she's usually up and dressed again within the hour. I'm at my wit's end." This woman's mother probably catnaps during the day and is therefore less tired at night. It makes sense to her, when she finds herself suddenly awake in bed and not at all sleepy, to assume it must be morning and time to get up.

"My husband used to be a dentist, a very brilliant man, with a gait like an eighteen-year-old," another woman recalls. "But he's starting to have trouble remembering words now, and his speech is not as fluid as it used to be. He's not the sweet, patient man he once was, either. He gets very angry, very unreasonable. He says things to me that he never would have said before." She knows how frustrating it must be to her husband, a man who loved words, when the words won't come—yet she's helpless to provide them for him.

"What am I supposed to do if he insists that he's going to visit his sister?" says another woman, also the wife of a man with Alzheimer's disease. "Should I tell him his sister died seven years ago? If I correct him, he just gets angry, and he forgets the next day what I told him anyway. Sometimes it's easier just to go along with him." It may be easier, say psychologists who work with Alzheimer's patients, but it is not fair to the individual to let him live in his delusions. Far better, for patient and family alike, to try a strategy of "gentle correction."

"I have no brothers or sisters, so my mother, who can't take care of herself, lives with me," another daughter of an Alzheimer's patient says. "She wouldn't give up her apartment, even when it was obvious she couldn't live alone anymore. We had to trick her into moving in with us by making her think she was just coming for Thanksgiving dinner. Now, she sometimes looks me straight in the eye and says—in a bitter, bitter voice that makes me want to run into another room and cry—'It would be nice if my daughter came to visit me once in a while.' " It's painful, she says, to love a mother who is not only dependent, but who cannot even recognize who it is she's dependent on.

To the casual observer—or even to the worried, loving family—the early stages of Alzheimer's disease often look like personality changes that are within the individual's control. Imagine the anger that could be generated by an old man or old woman who seems perfectly healthy yet who exhibits the symptoms of "early dementia" outlined by psychiatrist Eric Pfeiffer of the University of South Florida: "depression, listlessness, loss of interest, easy fatigability, lack of concentration, anxiety or agitation, . . . irritability, social withdrawal, emotional outburst, inconsiderateness, petulance, unaccustomed moral laxity, or irregular work attendance." How willful these symptoms seem, and how difficult it is to discern that they are caused by an underlying disease process affecting the brain.

Alzheimer's disease is not willfulness, is not stubbornness, is not insanity. It is neurological disease that is the fault of no one. It leads to behavior that is usually beyond the victim's control. And in that knowledge there is perhaps some relief for families that must watch their loved ones change.

Not Just the Old

In 1906 a patient of the German pathologist Alois Alzheimer died. She was fifty-five years old, and for the past four and a half years she had exhibited strange mental symptoms—memory loss, inability to reason, and profound overall intellectual deterioration. When his patient died, Alzheimer performed an autopsy of her brain, and there he found the two types of abnormal formations that are today considered the hallmarks of the disease named in his honor. Alzheimer published a paper theorizing that the brain lesions had caused his patient's unusual, rapid mental decay.

Within three years, the term "Alzheimer's disease" was being used to mean "pre-senile dementia," a condition that mimicked what were then the well-accepted changes of "senility," but which occurred in patients in their forties and fifties. The confirmation of the diagnosis of Alzheimer's disease, then as now, could only be made on autopsy, and could only be assured if the pathologist found the two types of abnormal formations typical of the disorder: neurofibrillary tangles and neuritic (also called agrophylic or senile) plaques.

For most of this century, a sharp distinction was made between Alzheimer's disease—"pre-senile dementia"—and "senile dementia." When persons in middle age began to lose their memories, act confused and disoriented, and show other signs of mental deterioration, their physicians, after proper neurological testing, were likely to diagnose the condition as Alzheimer's disease. But old people with the same symptoms were rarely given even the neurological testing, much less the diagnosis. Their problems, the doctors were sure, were due not to diseased brains but to diseased blood vessels, and were inevitable with age.

Beginning in the 1950s, the feeling began to spread that maybe the doctors were wrong. Part of the reason for this reappraisal was the scientific study being made of GIs killed in the Korean War, which showed that even young men had signs of the beginnings of atherosclerosis ("hardening of the arteries"), previously thought to be a disease of old age. As the notion faded that atherosclerosis was the inevitable result of age, the cavalier diagnosis of "cerebral atherosclerosis" ("hardening of the arteries of the brain") whenever an old person became forgetful or confused also began to be questioned.

At about this time, scientists were making a curious connection between "pre-senile" and "senile" dementia: they seemed to be the same disease that happened to strike people at different ages. This was a startling notion. But as it gained acceptance in the 1960s and 1970s, it removed some of the therapeutic nihilism that surrounded "senile dementia" in the past. It allowed scientists for the first time to believe that the disease, today called Alzheimer's disease even when it strikes people over sixty-five, was not inevitable with age but was a pathological process — a process with a distinct cause that someday could be found, treated, and cured.

Plaques and Tangles

The brain lesions characteristic of Alzheimer's disease — plaques and tangles — are the key to finding the cure. Researchers are now trying to piece together theories of where the abnormal lesions come from, how they interfere with mental functioning, and whether, once they occur, they can somehow be undone. Most scientists agree that the presence of these lesions in the brain, especially in the important regions in which they are found (such as the cerebral cortex and the hippocampus), is directly related to the mental changes of Alzheimer's disease. The Swiss researcher Jean Constantinidis is one of the scientists whose work helped lead to this conclusion. Constantinidis studied brain autopsies of 648 elderly individuals and divided them into seven groups according to the concentration of their brain lesions. The groups ranged from those with a high concentration of plaques and a very high concentration of tangles in the hippocampus and neocortex, to a control group of elderly patients with no plaques and no tangles whatsoever. He found that 355 persons fit into the three groups with the highest density of lesions, 221 into the three groups with the lowest density, and 72 into the control group with no lesions at all. The difference among the groups in terms of mental changes before death was striking. In the three most severely affected groups, 100 percent of the patients had shown signs of amnesia, beginning at an average age ranging from sixty-seven to seventy-six. In the three less severely affected groups, incidence of amnesia ranged from 72 to 87 percent, and its onset was much later, at about the age of seventy-nine. In the control group, who had no noticeable brain lesions, only 30 percent had shown signs of amnesia.

The lesions, then, seemed directly related to memory changes. Constantinidis found a similar pattern for the presence of what he calls "instrumental disorders"—loss of speech (aphasia), of previously acquired skills (apraxia), and of the ability to recognize the meaning of things heard, seen, felt, tasted, or smelled (agnosia). When plaques were present on autopsy and the density of neurofibrillary tangles in the neocortex was high, 91 percent of Constantinidis' subjects had exhibited these three instrumental disorders before they died. When the tangle density in the neocortex was moderate, the figure dropped to 65 percent, and to 51 percent when the density was low. When neurofibrillary tangles were found only in the hippocampus, not extending into the neocortex, only 32 percent had shown instrumental disorders, and when even the tangle density in the hippocampus was low, just 16 percent had. When plaques were present without tangles, instrumental disorders were seen in just 12 percent of the subjects, and in the control group, where no lesions were evident, instrumental disorders existed in just 3 percent. "Thus," Constantinidis concludes, "there is a correlation between the density and diffusion of neurofibrillary tangles (particularly in the neocortex) and the incidence of instrumental disorders."

These and other findings have led many scientists to believe that the plaques and tangles are the key to the mental changes of Alzheimer's disease. Therefore, in their search for an explanation of the disorder, the first question they have asked is: Just what are these lesions?

Neurofibrillary tangles and neuritic plaques are found to some degree in most very old brains. According to one Japanese study, nearly 99 percent of persons over the age of eighty have some plaques and some tangles. Most people, though, never develop *enough* of these lesions to lose memory and function. In Alzheimer's disease, the plaques and tangles occur in concentrations several times higher than the levels found in the healthy aged brain. And, perhaps more importantly, they tend to cluster in Alzheimer's disease in the brain regions with greatest impact on intellectual performance: the hippocampus, the frontal cortex, and the temporal cortex.

Neurofibrillary tangles, according to Dr. Robert Terry, chairman of pathology at the University of California at San Diego, appear to be made of two strands normally within the neuron, called filaments, that for some unknown reason wrap around each other into a spiral. Recent research indicates that the protein making up the filaments is abnormal—which could be the first step in finding a method for detecting the presence of tangles short of an autopsy of the brain. Dr. Dennis Selkoe, a neurologist at the Harvard Medical School, is hoping to identify the abnormal protein of neurofibrillary tangles, or perhaps an antibody that arises in the presence of this protein, to develop a definitive diagnostic test. Selkoe theorizes that the protein may arise from the process of cellular cross-linking, a process that has been associated with such age-related conditions as cataracts. He recently found that the same enzyme thought to be responsible for cross-linking in the lens of the eye—an enzyme called trans-glutaminase—is active in the brain as well.

Neurofibrillary tangles occur inside the brain cell. When they are found outside the cell, in the synapse, they usually are clustered with other degenerating cell components to form what is known as a neuritic plaque. At the core of each plaque is a mass of protein called amyloid which, Terry says, has no business being in the brain at all. Researchers are now trying to find out where the amyloid comes from.

Denham Harman, a chemist at the University of Nebraska School of Medicine, has hypothesized that amyloid may be formed by molecule fragments known as free radicals. Free radicals are highly reactive pieces of molecules in search of other molecules to link up with. In their hunt, they bombard an organism's cells and, according to Harman, may contribute not only to the development of neuritic plaques but also to the aging process as a whole. Vitamin E, he says, has been shown to counter the effects of free radicals.

Amyloid also contains high amounts of aluminum, leading some to theorize that high levels of the metal in the diet or the air may contribute to the formation of senile plaques. The aluminum theory has been bolstered by the work of Donald Crapper McLachlan, a psychologist at the

University of Toronto, who found that Alzheimer's disease patients had aluminum concentrations in their brains that were ten to thirty times the normal level. The areas of highest concentration, he found, were the areas where the plaques and tangles formed in greatest density: the hippocampus, frontal cortex, and temporal cortex. The current theory is that the underlying disease process somehow weakens the blood-brain barrier—which usually prevents environmental toxins from passing into the brain—and thus allows aluminum into regions of the brain where it can do damage. In this view, high concentrations of aluminum in the brain are a result, not a cause, of Alzheimer's disease.

Scientists' imaginations have been captured recently by the possibility of a viral or genetic link to Alzheimer's disease. Buoyed by the medical success stories of the last twenty years—the conquering of a host of viral diseases, such as polio, smallpox, rubella, and measles, and the control, through prenatal screening, of such genetic disorders as Down's syndrome and Tay-Sachs disease—scientists are hoping that Alzheimer's disease falls into one of these two categories. That would, they believe, make Alzheimer's a potentially curable, or preventable, illness—if only the key to its mystery can be found and turned.

Slow Viruses: The Alzheimer's Time Bomb?

Slow viruses may provide such a key. Slow, or latent, viruses are particular mysteries in the mysterious world of infectious agents. They are never seen, and they leave none of the hints of their presence—antibody formation, pus, and inflammation—that characterize most infections. Their presence can only be inferred from a knowledge of the route of transmission of the disease they cause. One especially remarkable case occurred in the early 1960s in Papua, New Guinea, where scores of tribal people were dying of a distinct brain illness known as kuru. The fatal disease caused uncontrollable tremors, total paralysis, and, finally, death, and was wildly epidemic among the Fore people of the remote New Guinean highlands. It seemed that kuru must be due to some sort of infectious agent, since it was so prevalent among the Fore but in no other group. But where was the agent? How was it spread? Neuroscientist D. Carleton Gajdusek of the National Institutes of Health (NIH), who won the 1976 Nobel Prize for his work in New Guinea, was the first to figure out the puzzle: the natives were cannibals, and part of their ritualistic funeral ceremony was eating the brains—and spreading the brains on their own bodies—of their diseased neighbors. The infectious agent was thus being transmitted directly from the victim of kuru to its next victim, because one was eating the other.

The pattern of transmission of Alzheimer's disease is now presenting a similar puzzle. Alzheimer's disease often occurs in familial clusters; in an estimated 10 to 15 percent of Alzheimer's cases, the illness seems to run in the family, and in those families a patient's children run a 50-50 chance of developing Alzheimer's disease. "But it's not just a simple genetic transmission," points out neurologist Robert Katzman. In identical twin pairs, he says, when one twin gets Alzheimer's disease, the other twin runs a 60 percent chance of developing it, too. Although this seems like a high risk, "it's about the same as the incidence of tuberculosis in two identical twins. If Alzheimer's disease were simply genetic, the incidence in twins would be 100 percent. So maybe the link between Alzheimer's disease and the families is not in the genes but in the environment, or the metabolism, or the psychosocial surroundings."

Since only about 10 to 15 percent of the cases of Alzheimer's disease qualify as "familial clusters," scientists believe that whatever it is that causes the clustering, be it genetic or environmental, probably cannot explain every isolated case of Alzheimer's disease. But the familial cases have led to some important discoveries in the search for a cause of the disease. For example, Gajdusek and his colleague at NIH, Clarence Gibbs, have injected bits of brain from patients who died of Alzheimer's disease into the brains of primates to see whether, as in the cannibals of New Guinea, the introduction of one brain piece into the system of another individual can carry with it the infectious agent, and thus transmit the disease. In two instances where the patient had died of the familial form of Alzheimer's disease (that is, when a close relative had also suffered from the same illness), the primates began to show signs of brain changes after receiving the injection. When injected parts of brains from Alzheimer's disease victims who had had no history of the illness in their families—the so-called random cases of Alzheimer's—the primate brains did not change at all. These findings are intriguing, but they still have not been replicated.

Genetic Theories

The biological detective work that has gone into the study of Alzheimer's disease has turned up some other theories as to its origin that are in many ways as intriguing as the slow virus theory. For instance, some pieces of evidence, quite apart from the familial clustering that can be explained by common exposure to an infectious agent, seem to point to a genetic cause of the disease.

One of the clearest signs that Alzheimer's disease may at least be related to the chromosomes—the carriers of genes, which in turn determine hereditary characteristics—is the story of Down's syndrome. Down's syndrome, a form of mental retardation that was once called "mongoloidism" because of the almond-shaped eyes of its victims, is caused by the presence of one extra chromosome. Because of an aberration in the formation of the egg, which ordinarily contributes one-half of a normal embryo's complement of forty-six chromosomes, the Down's syndrome baby receives an extra dose of chromosome #21 from its mother. Thus, he or she is born with forty-seven chromosomes (twenty-three from the father, twenty-four from the mother—the full complement plus a third chromosome on pair #21,) and the condition is known by scientists as trisomy 21.

Such aberrations in egg or sperm formation seem to happen fairly frequently, but usually the resulting trisomy embryo is so abnormal that it miscarries early in pregnancy. Trisomy 21 is different. The infant is born, but remains mentally retarded and often deficient in many other ways, frequently showing hearing problems, heart abnormalities, and other physical disorders. Because of the accompanying disabilities, persons with Down's syndrome have in the past rarely lived much beyond the age of twenty.

But advanced medical science has worked wonders with severely sick people, and victims of Down's syndrome have benefited along with numerous others of the chronically ill. Today Down's syndrome patients are living well into middle age, and physicians are for the first time witnessing a curious phenomenon: these people age prematurely. And one of the typical problems they encounter are the brain changes of Alzheimer's disease—great densities of neurofibrillary tangles and neuritic plaques.

Because "dementia" is defined as the loss of mental capabilities previously achieved, it cannot be applied to mentally retarded individuals who never achieved what is considered "normal" mental functioning. These Down's syndrome patients, then, do not really have Alzheimer's disease in the strictest sense. But something seems to happen to their brains that, while perhaps not evident clinically, is easily detectable when an autopsy is performed after they have died. Scientists are now studying the formation carried on chromosome #21 to see why the presence of an extra chromosome would seem to cause the development of plaques and tangles.

Leonard Heston, a psychiatrist at the University of Minnesota, has done extensive studies on the genetic component of Alzheimer's disease—and he keeps coming back to the link to Down's syndrome. The development of plaques and tangles in the brains of Down's patients past middle age, he says, may be part of the general acceleration of aging that has been observed in Down's syndrome, in which persons exhibit premature "graying and hair loss, pigment deposition in skin, cataracts, occlusive vascular disease, diabetes, and immune system changes." Another possibility is that the same chromosome responsible for Down's syndrome—chromosome #21—is also somehow responsible for Alzheimer's disease.

Persons with Alzheimer's disease of early onset, Heston has found, run a risk of having Down's syndrome in the family that is four times higher than normal. And they run a higher than normal risk of having blood and lymph cancers in the family, such as lymphocytic leukemia, Hodgkin's disease, and lymphosarcoma—cancers that also occur at above-average rates in the families of persons with Down's syndrome.

These familial clusterings are most profound in families in which Alzheimer's disease appears early in the patient's life. Of the 125 Alzheimer's patients Heston studied, 56 had an early onset, and their first-degree relatives (parents, children, and siblings) ran a risk of developing Alzheimer's that was ten to twenty times greater than the risk of the general population. Interestingly, the familial risks were concentrated in less than half of the families studied, leading Heston and others to think that there might be two kinds of Alzheimer's disease—familial Alzheimer's and randomly occurring Alzheimer's.

Other associations between Alzheimer's and Down's syndrome have also been made. Some of them are unconfirmed, but they are nonetheless intriguing. One scientist found that fingerprint patterns in Alzheimer's patients were similar to those found in Down's patients. Another found that persons with Alzheimer's disease were significantly more likely to have been born to mothers over the age of thirty-five—an association that has been well established as a risk factor of Down's syndrome.

The current thinking among geneticists is that a predisposition for Alzheimer's disease is carried on several genes, and that the disease has a "variable, age-related penetrance" —that is, a tendency to reveal itself late in life if exposed to the appropriate toxins, infectious agents, or lifestyles. Jean Constantinidis of the University of Geneva has turned this notion around somewhat, theorizing that the trait for Alzheimer's disease is carried on a single dominant gene that is influenced by several inhibitor genes. If one or more inhibitor gene is present, he says, the disease will not develop until quite late in life. In the absence of any inhibitor genes, however, Alzheimer's disease strikes in middle age.

The Choline Connection

In 1976 three groups of British scientists, working independently, made a dramatic discovery about the brain chemistry of Alzheimer's disease: All of the patients they studied almost totally lacked the brain enzyme needed to make the neurotransmitter involved in thought and memory. Peter Davies at the Medical Research Council of Edinburgh, David Bowen of the Institute of Neurology in London, and Elaine Perry at the University of Newcastle all found a remarkable decline in the amount of the enzyme choline acetyltransferase in certain regions of the brain's cortex—most prominently, in the hippocampus. Choline acetyltransferase is known as a "biosynthetic enzyme" for the neurotransmitter acetycholine; without it, no acetylcholine can be manufactured. And without acetylcholine, nothing can be remembered or learned.

According to Peter Davies, who is now at Albert Einstein College of Medicine in New York, the amount of choline acetyltransferase in the hippocampus of persons with Alzheimer's disease is reduced by an average of 91.2 percent compared to the enzyme level in the brains of normal old people. Although the enzyme level is known to decline gradually with age—so that a ninety-five-year-old has lost as much as 70 percent of his choline acetyltransferase in the course of adulthood—it generally is not missed. But the even larger fall-off found in Alzheimer's disease could account for some behavioral changes that are not found in normal aging.

"It appears that a person can drop to 20 percent of the young adult level without harm," Davies said in a New York *Times* article shortly after moving to the United States, "but the next 5 percent is likely to cause serious trouble."

Significantly, the drop in choline acetyltransferase levels in Alzheimer's disease is most striking in the two areas of the brain where plaques and tangles accumulate — the cortex and the hippocampus. There seems to be a direct connection between a loss of choline acetyltransferase and the development of neuritic plaques, since the less choline acetyltransferase an individual has, the more plaques in his brain. A similar relationship has been noted between the decline in choline acetyltransferase and performance on intelligence tests: that is, the less of the enzyme (and, by inference, the neurotransmitter acetylcholine) an individual has, the more impaired his memory and thinking abilities. Scientists next must try to determine in which direction these relationships occur. Does the loss of choline acetyltransferase cause plaque formation, or vice versa?

During the 1980s brain researchers found that other neurotransmitter systems also were compromised or debilitated in Alzheimer's disease patients. They found that the brain cell region responsible for the production of the noradrenergic transmitters exhibits significant cell loss in Alzheimer's disease. This region, the locus ceruleus, is the site of origin for noradrenaline, also called norepinephrine. Noradrenaline is the "fight or flight hormone" that seems to be reduced in about one-half of the patients with Alzheimer's disease.

Another neurotransmitter, somatostatin, also is significantly reduced in Alzheimer's disease. Researchers have found a 50 percent to 90 percent reduction of somatostatin in the cerebral cortex of Alzheimer's disease patients. They are not sure what role somatostatin plays, but they have noted that it coexists in brain cells where acetylcholine is found. Reduced levels of somatostatin are known to accompany depression and the active stages of multiple sclerosis; increased levels have been noted in patients with Huntington's disease.

130

The fact that more than one neurotransmitter probably is involved in Alzheimer's disease helps explain the disappointing results clinicians have had with trying to boost only acetylcholine. "Even when the acetylcholine levels are increased, the somatostatin levels remain miserably low," says Suzanne Corkin, a psychologist at the Massachusetts Institute of Technology. "But it is hard to get the FDA to approve research in which more than one transmitter at a time is supplemented." Corkin envisions a day when an Alzheimer's patient can take a "cocktail" of several neurotransmitters to raise the levels of all brain chemicals that are depleted by the disease.

Diagnosing the Disease

A definitive diagnosis of Alzheimer's disease cannot easily be made while a person is alive. No matter how suggestive the mental symptoms are, the physician cannot be absolutely sure that they are due to Alzheimer's disease until he or she sees the plaques and tangles under the microscope—and this cannot occur until the patient has died and the brain is examined on autopsy. Recently, the NIA issued a set of guidelines to aid in the post-mortem diagnosis of Alzheimer's disease based on the amount of lesions that could be detected on brain autopsy. NIA concluded that a pathologist could make a definitive diagnosis of Alzheimer's disease, even with no knowledge of the patient's clinical history, if he or she could find the following numbers of brain lesions in each microscopic field of 1 square millimeter of tissue:

> In a patient aged fifty or less: two to five plaques and two to five tangles per field.
>
> In a patient aged fifty to sixty-five: eight plaques per field and some tangles.

In a patient aged sixty-six to seventy-five: ten plaques per field and some tangles.

In a patient aged seventy-five or more: fifteen plaques per field and some tangles.

If the pathologist knows that the patient also exhibited symptoms of dementia prior to death, a definitive diagnosis of Alzheimer's disease could be made with only half as many lesions per brain sample.

There are, however, several clinical tests that can be performed that are helpful in the diagnosis of Alzheimer's disease, allowing patients and their families a generally good idea of what they can expect in the last few years of life.

When an elderly patient comes to the doctor with symptoms of intellectual deterioration, of course, the first thing the doctor should do is rule out a treatable cause for the problem—drug intoxication, metabolic or endocrine disorder, depression, infection, or any of the 100 or so reversible disorders described in the previous chapter. Once these possibilities have been eliminated, the physician is generally advised to wait about six to nine months before attempting a firm diagnosis. Since Alzheimer's disease is always progressive, some changes in mental function can be expected to have occurred between the first and second visits; if the patient has not become more confused and more forgetful in the space of half a year, it is possible the patient does not have Alzheimer's disease.

If his or her condition has worsened, though, certain tests may help shed light on the cause of the problem. The electroencephalogram, which monitors electrical activity in the brain ("brain waves") through electrodes attached to the scalp and forehead, often appears in an irregular pattern in Alzheimer's disease. The activity becomes markedly slower in certain regions of the brain, causing a reduction in the height of the brain wave spikes and a greater distance from one peak to the next.

The computed tomography (CT) scan, which scans the brain in slices and creates a three-dimensional picture with the aid of a computer, can also be used to help suggest the diagnosis of Alzheimer's disease. The CT scan of an Alzheimer's patient usually reveals atrophy, or shrinkage, in the temporal lobes of the brain, and an enlargement of the large fluid-filled spaces within the lobes, called the ventricles. Ventricular enlargement and temporal lobe atrophy do not mean Alzheimer's disease, scientists are quick to point out; they simply are consistent with the diagnosis. In other words, if a patient shows these changes on a CT scan, he might have Alzheimer's; if he does not, he probably doesn't (although a few patients with Alzheimer's disease do have normal CT scans). The prime value of a CT scan is its ability to rule out other, possibly treatable causes of the dementia.

Scientists are now studying an even more sophisticated computerized brain scan device called the positron emission tomogram (PET) to see whether it produces patterns characteristic of Alzheimer's disease. In PET, the subject is given an isotope, or radioactive form, of glucose, the chemical that is metabolized by the body primarily in the brain. (The brain, which makes up about 2 percent of an individual's weight, utilizes 40 percent of the glucose that passes through the body.) PET picks up the emissions of the isotope as the brain metabolizes it, detecting 10,000 to 15,000 separate bits of information over the course of several hours and then compiling them all, by computer, into a picture of glucose utilization. Early indications are that the typical Alzheimer's brain shows greatly reduced cerebral metabolism in a PET scan. The use of this procedure is still in its infancy, but some doctors hope it will eventually provide a better picture of the brain than even the CT scan. The CT scan delineates anatomical, or structural, changes; the PET scan is capable of showing changes in glucose utilization—the brain in action—and thus might be even more helpful in diagnosing and treating neurological disease.

PET's potential was demonstrated in 1983 by Mony de Leon and his colleagues at New York University. De Leon examined eight patients with Alzheimer's disease and eleven controls, and found that their CT scans were virtually indistinguishable. But when he compared PET scans, the Alzheimer's patients revealed a reduction in glucose metabolism of 21 to 28 percent. PET scanning has also proved useful in differentiating Alzheimer's disease from other common causes of dementia, such as multi-infarct dementia and Huntington's disease, that reveal different patterns of metabolic derangement in the brain.

Among the newer imaging techniques that may also prove useful in the diagnosis of Alzheimer's disease are SPECT (single photon emission computed tomography) and NMR (nuclear magnetic resonance). SPECT operates along the same lines as PET, but with a difference: instead of using a positron, a subatomic particle that must be generated by a multimillion-dollar piece of equipment called a cyclotron housed in a nearby major university, it uses a photon, a subatomic particle that can be made available to the smallest community hospital because of its long shelf life. NMR, like CT, delineates brain anatomy, but it uses radio frequency waves in a strong magnetic field rather than the potentially harmful ionizing radiation used in the CT scan. A group of Scottish researchers reported in 1983 that they could differentiate Alzheimer's patients from patients with multi-infarct dementia based on NMR measurements in the white matter of the brain. "None of the current tomographic imaging techniques—CT, PET, SPECT, or NMR—yet provides a reliable diagnostic test for dementia," notes Dr. Marvin B. Cohen, a professor of radiology at the University of California at Los Angeles. "However, progress is being made in each, and such a test may well be available in the next few years."

Coping Strategies

Like other diseases affecting the brain, Alzheimer's disease changes the victim's personality. Because it makes people seem lazy and uncooperative, and because it destroys the very qualities that make them uniquely themselves, Alzheimer's disease creates a special kind of terror. "You wouldn't be reacting this way if you had been told your mother had cancer," chided one expert on the disease, Katherine Bick of the National Institutes of Health, when the daughter of an Alzheimer's patient became "hysterical" over her mother's diagnosis. And yet, Bick said later, she understood this woman's intense fears. "The thought of her mother's brain, her whole identity, changing—well, that's different, somehow, from the thought of her body being destroyed."

In the early stages of Alzheimer's disease many individuals are able to cover up for the loss of memory and orientation caused by the neurological changes. "My mother is smart enough still that she will say nothing unless asked a direct question," said one New Jersey woman at a meeting of an Alzheimer's disease family support group. "And then she will answer in as few words as possible. She doesn't want to let on that she keeps forgetting the words she wants to use. It's almost a slyness."

Unfortunately, there are moments of clarity during the early stages of dementia, times in which the patients somehow understand that they are losing their grip on the world. These times can be profoundly depressing for victims and families alike. Perhaps it is helpful to know that the clarity will eventually disappear, and the Alzheimer's patients, though never again to possess the mental powers they once had, can at least be made to feel comfortable, at ease, and content.

As the disease progresses, and patients become more and more incapable of thinking in abstract terms, remembering, or expressing themselves, they may continue to develop tricks to avoid placing themselves in revealing situations. If asked a direct question ("How old are you, Mrs. Collins?") they deflect a direct answer that might give away their ignorance ("How old do you think I am?" if Mrs. Collins is basically a friendly woman, or perhaps, "What business is it of yours?" if she is not). Other patients with Alzheimer's disease invent elaborate answers bearing little relation to reality or to the original question—a trick psychiatrists call "confabulation." (This works especially well if the story is one whose truthfulness the questioner cannot check: "How old am I? I was born in Ohio, but we moved to Nebraska when I was small. My mother was only seventeen when she had me, and she was only nineteen when she had my brother. She was a pretty woman, but my father treated her badly . . .") Some patients may deny that anything is wrong with their memory or ability to think. ("What's all the fuss about? Why don't you stop asking me all these questions and just let me go home?") And some patients may engage in another defensive trick called "perseveration."

An individual who perseverates, as Florida psychiatrist Eric Pfeiffer explains, returns over and over again during an interview to the first answer, the first story, the first word that had been right or nearly right, and tries to stick with it in hopes of it being right again. Thus, one of Pfeiffer's patients, who had been given a Rorschach Inkblot Test, identified the first design as "a Christmas tree decoration," and went on to call every other inkblot she was shown "a Christmas tree." And an old man who was asked to copy the sentence "Now is the time for all good men to come to the aid of their party" wrote the following, also typical of perseveration: "Now is the time time t t t t . . ." until the "t's" trailed off the page.

"The presence of such defensive maneuvers indicates two things," Pfeiffer says. "[First,] the intellectual deficit has been present for some considerable period of time, six months at a minimum, more likely a year or longer; [second,] the ego is not overwhelmed by the deficit but is still trying to cope with it."

Consider this eighty-year-old British violinist, a gracious woman whose brain disease rendered her incapable of remembering events for more than a few minutes. She had successfully avoided giving herself away through the judicious use of notebooks and her well ingrained social skills, which guided her through her dealings with other people. Yet the ruse could not last forever. As Sir Martin Roth, a psychiatrist at Cambridge University in England, describes it:

> *One evening she was performing a difficult and intricate Beethoven quartet with musical friends. At the end of the performance, there was a brief pause. The enthusiasm of the cellist had been ignited. He pleaded that they should play just one more work. The eighty-year-old lady, who had played immaculately in the previous performance (drawing on long-established skill and knowledge), proposed that they play the Beethoven Opus 59 No. 1 Quartet. Her friends gazed*

at her in complete astonishment. "Why," remonstrated one of them, "we just finished playing that."

This woman did not have Alzheimer's disease, but she is mentioned here as a reminder of the highly idiosyncratic nature of dementia in old age. The rate at which individuals decline is highly varied, as is the sequence in which various functions are lost. But, perhaps most important, something still remains—in this woman's case, her remarkable musical skill. The most valuable thing that can be done for persons with Alzheimer's disease is to find those functions that remain, be it the ability to knit or sing or mow the lawn or walk the dog, and to encourage them to use those skills for as long as possible.

The following chapter will describe a patient whose family now is wrestling with the problem of how many of his remaining functions to take away from him. Stanley Scott still works in the family-owned business, still drives his car and the company pickup truck, and still operates a crane at work. But his memory loss is profound, and the disease has made him violent. When is it time to tell Stanley Scott that his mistakes are costing money, and that his temper makes it dangerous for him to operate heavy machinery? And what will happen to him when he is told?

⟡ **6** ⟡

Alzheimer's Disease: The Scotts' Story

The autumn sun streaming into Bertha Scott's bedroom woke her just before the alarm did, and she marveled at its warmth. Suddenly the buzzer went off, and her husband, Stanley, was awake and out of bed in a flash. It was a Sunday in October and Stanley was, as always, dressed within minutes.

Feeling lazy—an uncommon luxury for her—Bertha, on a whim, asked a favor of Stanley. "I feel like being waited on this morning," she said to him, revealing the gap between her two front teeth when she smiled. "Do you think you could bring me a cup of instant coffee?"

Stanley, a quiet man, headed silently for the kitchen, while Bertha arranged her plumpish body on the bedclothes and gazed out the window. Within minutes, Stanley had returned. "What's instant coffee?" he asked.

The reverie brought on by the morning sun was just ten minutes old, but Stanley already had shattered it. His question brought back to Bertha the nagging in the pit of her stomach that has not dissipated for seven years: Stanley has Alzheimer's disease. Stanley cannot remember things. Stanley is no longer like a husband, he is like a child.

Alzheimer's disease, we have seen, affects more than 2 million Americans, the majority of them over sixty-five. The doctors tell us that Alzheimer's disease produces "senile symptoms": memory loss, inability to calculate, poor judgment, irrationality, emotional outbursts, and often, in its later stages, inability to recognize family and friends, to control one's urine and bowel functions, to maintain personal hygiene, and, at the very end, even to remember one's own name. But hearing the professionals' recounting of symptoms is not the same as watching those symptoms in action, observing how they can change a man's personality and sully his relationship with his wife, his sons, and his brothers and sisters. For this reason, we shall meet Stanley Scott (the names of the family have been changed at their request) and, through Bertha and the rest of the Scott family, as well as through Stanley's psychotherapist and neurologist, we shall see exactly what it is like to live with Alzheimer's disease.

"Walking on Eggs": Stanley and Bertha

At fifty-eight, Stanley Scott is a relatively young victim of Alzheimer's, the incidence of which increases steadily with age and is highest between the ages of seventy and ninety. He is a trim man, his black hair graying only slightly at the temples, a smile on his face when he meets a doctor or a writer he wants to impress. But he smiles less often these days, and Bertha says he seems not to find joy in anything except his job. After thirty years of operating a crane for various construction companies in the exurbs of Philadelphia, Stanley went into partnership with his younger son, Steven, in 1974. The two men bought a junkyard in Bucks County, and Stanley set to work on the crane again, this time smashing cars instead of building houses.

His youthful appearance makes Stanley's erratic behavior and unreliable memory seem all the more bizarre. "Sometimes when he gets dressed up and you look at him," says his wife, "you just can't imagine that there's a thing wrong." And she's right: Stanley does look fit and healthy, and he seems at first meeting to be capable of carrying on an ordinary, casual conversation. But the pale eyes don't sparkle; within minutes of initial contact they have faded into the distance, and Stanley is no longer listening.

"He's awful quiet now," says Bertha, who is fifty-seven and dresses in the smart tailored clothes more typical of a career woman in town (which she is not) than of the wife of a farm boy–turned–crane operator (which she is). Her strawberry blond hair is tailored, too, and the only hints that she lives under stress come out in her strained, high voice and in her nervous munching of any food set before her. "If we go to a party or a cookout, he sits alone, and he doesn't very often get in on the conversation. Or he'll come sit with the women, alongside of me, and I'm just so glad to get to where there are some women to talk to. . . . When there's only a group of men around, he'll play with the kids, or he'll play with the dog. It's like he's not paying attention to the men."

Stanley's memory loss, which began about 1972, is profound. He cannot recognize old co-workers and neighbors; when he and Bertha run into people who lived near the farm on which he spent his first twenty-one years, he draws a total blank. He is beginning to have trouble keeping track of his nieces and nephews, the offspring of his nine brothers and sisters, six of whom still live a short drive from Stanley's home. And now he is forgetting, too, the tasks that have been second nature to him for a lifetime — simple tasks, like changing a tire. In the junkyard, one of his chores is to remove motors and other parts from the cars so they can be salvaged; he could do this easily two years ago, but he cannot now. "If they tell me to go out there and take a part off the car," he told Bertha in a rare moment of self-revelation, "I'm lost, I don't know what to do."

His forgetfulness comes out in other ways, too. "Thursday I went up to the yard," Bertha says, "and they asked him for the money he had collected on Wednesday night. [Another of Stanley's jobs is to deliver parts to customers and to collect payments from them.] He didn't have any money. He should have had fifty-five dollars; he didn't have any. He had money in his wallet, but he said it was all his money. I said, "Stanley, are you sure you had all that money in your wallet before?' He said, 'Well, I had a lot of money,' but he didn't remember how much money he really had. So then they got on the phone and they called the customers where he delivered — and they are the customers who always pay in cash. They all said, 'Yes, we paid him.' This morning, Saturday, he was all upset again, looking through his wallet. He said he had delivered some more parts last evening, and he said, 'I'm trying to find that money I got last night, because I don't want that to happen again. You were up there when it happened, when I couldn't find the money.' " Stanley's psychologist has urged him to keep a separate wallet for his collections, or to record payments in a notebook, or to carry a clipboard where he can clip the bill and the cash together. But Bertha says he shrugs off all suggestions. "He will not have anybody tell him what to do."

His refusal to change his life to adjust for his forgetfulness is a matter of stubbornness, not denial. Stanley has never denied that he is losing his memory. "I'm going just like my father," he has been muttering off and on to himself and to Bertha for the past seven years. "My father couldn't remember nothing, and I'm going the same way as my father."

Bertha remembers "Pop Scott" in his last years, and she says Stanley is indeed following in his footsteps. "Pop Scott got to the point where he didn't know me, he didn't even know his own sons or his own daughters. He didn't know anybody. You'd walk into the house and he'd say, 'Who are you?' I can remember, when Stanley was in the service and I was living at the farm, at dinnertime things would be put on the table and Pop Scott wouldn't know what they were. Now Stanley's the same way. He'll ask me, 'What's this? Have we ever had this before?' if I give him something like cranberry sauce. And sometimes I'll give him applesauce for a vegetable, and he'll say, 'Shall I eat this now, or is this dessert?' Each time he says one of those things, you kind of feel like you're in shock. And yet he doesn't see why you should worry about it."

Bertha was intimately involved in Pop Scott's illness, which lasted from his early fifties until his death at age sixty-two. Her mother-in-law, a lazy woman, called Bertha whenever there was a problem: if Pop Scott wet his pants, or "did his business" in a corner of the living room instead of the bathroom, she would call Bertha and ask her to come clean up. Bertha always did. She also went along on doctor visits to help dress and undress Pop Scott. "He wouldn't even know how," she remembers. "He'd wear this long underwear, and he wouldn't even know how to get his legs into them." For some reason, Mom Scott always sat outside in the waiting room during these sessions.

Bertha is not afraid of what Alzheimer's disease might do to Stanley in his later years; she has already nursed his father through *his* final stages. She is not afraid, but she dreads it. "When I see things that he does that his father did, for the next couple of days I can't think of nothing else," she admits. "Like one Sunday morning this summer, I went in to the bedroom and he's there cussing, 'I don't know what's wrong with this shirt.' And there he is, trying to put on my blouse."

When he watches television, Stanley also reminds Bertha of his father. "When his father was alive, they had a lot of musical variety shows on," she says, "and Pop Scott would watch the people dancing around in costumes and say, 'They're making goddamn fools of themselves.' Now, when a comedy program comes on, I love to sit and watch it, but Stanley doesn't know what I'm laughing at. He just says, 'Goddamn stupid fools.' That's the same thing his father said." Anything more complicated than the "Tic Tac Dough" game show, Bertha says, is too complicated for Stanley to follow. If he is watching a show with a story line, he seems to lose its continuity each time the camera angle shifts. So he does not watch television, and he does not go to the movies, and he does not listen to music. Instead, he goes to sleep.

"He goes to bed every night at seven or seven-thirty," she says. Each evening the routine is the same: "He would come home from work so mad! He'd walk into that house and I'd say, 'Hello, what kind of a day did you have? What did you do today?' No answer. He'd just go to the refrigerator, grab a can of beer, and go out and sit on the patio. He'd sit there till I would say, 'Dinner's ready.' He'd come in and eat dinner, then maybe I'd go outside, and he'd get up, get a bath, and go to bed. And that would be the night."

Once, gingerly, Bertha tried to suggest a change in the routine. "It gets so lonely sitting here night after night," she said as Stanley stood up to get ready for bed. "Can't you sit up with me for a little while?" The request, innocent as it seemed, set Stanley off into what Bertha calls "one of his fits"—temper tantrums she says he rarely displayed when he was younger. He yelled, he steamed, and finally he sat on the couch in stony silence, refusing to look at the television or to talk or gesture. Finally, by eight o'clock, Bertha begged Stanley to go to bed and leave her in peace. But he had his way. He didn't budge until eight-thirty. And Bertha never again asked for his company.

The "fits" are perhaps the hardest part of Alzheimer's disease for Bertha. Although the tantrums have eased somewhat in the five months that Stanley has been taking tranquilizers, Bertha is still living "on my edge. I'm waiting for him to do something and I don't know what he's going to do. If I say something to try to help him out I don't know how he's going to take it, if it's going to put him in one of his fits." The simplest thing can set him off: the suggestion that Stanley is mowing the grass badly, or that they should have a Sunday breakfast at home for a change instead of going, bright and early, to the same diner week after week.

So far Stanley has not hit Bertha, even in his wildest rages. Instead he bounces on furniture, punches doors and walls, yells and cries. But if they are in the car when Bertha says something that angers him, Stanley has been known to drive off the road, threatening to smash the car and kill them both. "He talks about killing himself a lot," Bertha says, "and I think he might do it in a fit of temper without really thinking about it, either by driving his car into a telephone pole or by shooting himself. . . . Every once in a while he gets out that .22 to see if it still fires."

In the middle of a fit of temper, Bertha says, her husband looks like a madman. She has been spared the sight for nearly six months now that she has learned to "walk on eggs" around Stanley. But his "fits" at the junkyard are becoming more and more frequent. "He took his fist one day up there when something went wrong," she says, "and he banged his fist until he bent the whole hood in on a car. He came home with his hands all swollen. I said, 'What's the matter with your hands?' 'Nothing.' The next day, we were having breakfast and he said to me, 'Look at my hands. Look how swollen they are. I wonder what happened.' He didn't remember what he had done the day before to make his hands swollen like that."

Bertha believes Stanley is inexpressibly sad. She says his work at the junkyard is the only thing that interests him anymore, the only thing that keeps him going. And even that seems to be slipping away from him. "To be perfectly honest, I don't think there's much he can do up there anymore," she says, "but I don't know how to tell him." She knows that he and his son Steve fight constantly about the way things should be run at the yard—especially now that Steve has decided to build an automatic crusher that will be able to do the work of Stanley and his thirty-five-year-old crane. The idea that the crusher will replace him—even though Steve wants his father to run the machine—has made Stanley "miserable," Bertha says, and she does not know what he would do if the crusher did in fact render Stanley obsolete. "I've told Stevie and told Stevie, 'I know you can't let him have his own way up at that junkyard, because he doesn't know sometimes the way he wants to do things. But as long as he could get his own way, there wouldn't be any problems at all.' I don't have too many problems if I just let him have his own way."

Stanley is aware that he can no longer smash cars or salvage parts or even collect payments with any reliability. "Every single night he looks in the want ads," his wife says. "But he could never work for anybody; he couldn't remember what he'd have to do. If they told him in the morning to do two or three jobs, he couldn't remember which ones he'd done. He could get a job as a janitor, but he couldn't remember which day he cleaned this room and which day he cleaned that room. He just couldn't work for anybody else." But, being the kind of man he is, with no interests outside of his job and no sense of self-worth if he is not working, Stanley couldn't *not* work, either.

Sometimes, Bertha says, Stanley talks about retiring—but she does not think he means it. "He says he's worked so hard all his life, and he says if he's going to die before he's sixty-five anyway he might as well be home these last couple of years and just enjoy himself. But he wouldn't enjoy himself. I'm afraid if he were home he'd just lie on the couch and sleep all day."

Nothing much can help Stanley anymore—and he seems, at times, to know it. Every time he goes to a new doctor, he embarrasses his wife by saying, "Take my brains out. Just take my brains out and see what's wrong with me." When his forgetfulness was diagnosed as cerebral arteriosclerosis in 1973—a common mistake at that time—Stanley was placed on a low-cholesterol diet that he followed almost religiously. He was delighted, says Bertha, at the thought that he could do something simple to forestall reliving his father's fate. Now, his neurologist has prescribed eight teaspoons a day of the dietary substance lecithin to try to improve Stanley's memory. (The theory is that lecithin, a precursor of the neurotransmitter acetylcholine, may stimulate production of acetylcholine, which is often all but absent in patients with Alzheimer's disease.) While Bertha sees no change, Stanley is certain that the lecithin will cure him. He eats the grainy stuff without complaint, sprinkling it on his cereal and in his juice eagerly, telling Bertha and Steve that he can feel himself getting better. Stanley does not like going to the psychotherapist, Bertha explains; he doesn't know what good talking will do. But now that his neurologist has given him lecithin, he doesn't mind his visits there. "If you could just give him a bag of pills," Bertha says to a writer whom Stanley is hesitant to meet, "he'd be down here in a flash."

Watching Stanley's optimism about a cure has been hard for Bertha, as she's become more and more convinced that a cure is out of their reach. She takes Stanley to the doctors, and has enrolled him in a federal study conducted at the University of Pennsylvania, not because she thinks it will help Stanley, but because she thinks that finding a cure for Alzheimer's disease might someday help her two sons, who she worries may also develop Alzheimer's disease when *they* reach middle age. "I'll take him anywhere," she says, "so long as there's something I can do that will help Lennie and Stevie. My biggest fear is that this is going to be repeated a third time."

Meanwhile, Bertha will feed Stanley his lecithin, and, if the need arises, will help him dress and eat and use the bathroom. "I've made enough trips to the state hospital," she says, remembering her own alcoholic father's last years at Norristown State, "that to clean up somebody's wet pants wouldn't bother me at all" if it meant keeping him out of there. The only time Bertha feels sorry for herself is when she talks to her friends who have intact, active husbands. "Sometimes I'll talk to Marge and she'll say, 'John is gonna help me polish the brass,' or 'John doesn't think I should move the sofa.' Stanley doesn't give one hoot what I do in that house. . . . It's pretty much like living alone now." And, she adds delicately, Stanley "just doesn't show me any more affection. He never kisses you good night or good morning. Nothing. Never touches you. Nothing."

As she muses about her life with her husband, Bertha

says carefully, "Stanley doesn't even think that he's doing anything wrong. Well, it really isn't that he's doing anything wrong; he can't help himself. But with his forgetting, like the day he was standing in the middle of the bedroom floor and holding his sport coat and said to me, 'What do I do with this?' when the closet's right there, these things just make knots or something go around in my stomach. And he doesn't see why any of this stuff that he does like this should upset me. If you say anything when he puts things on backward and he can't do anything—well, I just hate to tell him when he does something wrong. I try to hide it when I get upset; I don't want to make him feel any worse than what he feels."

If she had known about Alzheimer's disease when she was younger, Bertha says without blinking an eye, "I would never have gotten into the Scott family." It is the only time she raises her voice.

The Alzheimer's Legacy: Leonard and Linda

"Dad was always saying the Scotts' brains were no good," says Leonard Scott, at thirty-five the elder of Stanley's two sons. "I hope to God he's wrong," adds Leonard's wife, Linda. The physical resemblance between Leonard and his father is uncanny: when Leonard looks at Stanley, he must feel as though he is seeing his own face in twenty years. Will Leonard's face, too, become as gloomy, as distant? "One of the reasons I married Lennie is that I thought he was just like his father, and I thought his father was so neat," Linda says. "I thought if he turned out just like his father, that would suit me fine for a husband." Today, Linda reads voraciously about Alzheimer's disease to arm herself against the fate she had so blithely hoped for fifteen years earlier. She accompanies her in-laws on their monthly treks to the University of Pennsylvania, takes an active role in trying to coax other family members to go down to the university for testing, listens to Bertha's stories, and worries. The more she learns about Alzheimer's disease, she says, the better she can cope with whatever awaits her and Leonard—and their two little girls.

The tendency to develop Alzheimer's disease is generally thought to be inherited, especially in a family in which it appears over several generations. But the trait, most scientists feel, is one with "incomplete penetrance"—that is, even if an individual carries the tendency, any number of nongenetic factors can come into play to determine whether or not the potential for Alzheimer's disease ever manifests itself. And the "polygenic" nature makes predictions of inheritance of Alzheimer's disease all but impossible. Once an individual develops other kinds of genetic disease—say, Huntington's disease—doctors know precisely what his gene makeup is: it includes the single gene that carries the Huntington's trait. Then they know that each of the patient's offspring runs a 50 percent chance of inheriting that single gene. But Alzheimer's disease is wholly unpredictable, because it is found not on one but probably on several genes, and the information on those genes is not a definitive sentence of Alzheimer's, but only a tendency toward it.

The uncertainty of the pattern of inheritance of Alzheimer's disease is what so worries Leonard and Linda.

The only college graduate in the Scott family, Linda Scott is a home economics teacher, antiques collector, and aspiring writer. She is a slim woman with blond, country good looks, who seems to run on cigarettes and enthusiasm, and she can talk nonstop. "I deal with things much better when they're out front, even when they're awful," she says.

Her husband's approach is different. "I try not to dwell on it," says Leonard, a soft-spoken, even-tempered man who drives a tractor-trailer, lives in a house he built himself, and helps Linda with the dishes and chores when he is home. "If it's gonna happen it's gonna happen. But I'm more than willing to cooperate with anybody to try to find out if it's going to happen to me or if there's anything that can be done about it."

"I'm not so worried about it happening," Linda says, "or that I couldn't face it if it happened. That doesn't bother me."

From Leonard: "Maybe it would change our lives if we *knew* it was going to happen. Maybe you'd mortgage the ranch and go out and have a good time now, because later on—that's not going to be part of it then."

From Linda: "But if you don't worry about it, maybe you don't do something about it. That's my attitude."

And Leonard, tired of the subject: "But what can you do about it? There's nothing you can do about it."

Linda overflows with ideas about what she can do about it. She says she continually is thwarted at the University of Pennsylvania, where Stanley has been part of a federal "case-control study" of Alzheimer's disease. She offers theories and suggestions regarding Stanley and Leonard, she says, and is made to feel as though she is interfering with the design of the scientists' epidemiological research. "At the very beginning, I had done some reading about this lecithin that they've been giving people," she says. "I asked at University Hospital about whether there was any treatment like that for Dad; I realized they were just trying to determine cause in their study, but was there any treatment? I said I'd been doing some reading on vitamins and things like that. The doctor just said, 'Oh, no, none of that's legal in the United States. They're only doing that in Europe, ma'am.' So I went to the health food store and just bought some lecithin anyway. From what I'd been reading, even for normal people it did not hurt within a certain dosage to take it. So Lennie and I started taking it. Then I read something else that said too little might almost be as harmful as too much, so then I thought that maybe neither of us should really be taking it; I really could be bollixing it up. I asked the doctors about that, and again, no answer. Then I couldn't go with Mom one time, and when she came home, that's what they had put Dad on that day! It made me mad that when I first brought it up, they wouldn't say, 'We're going to consider lecithin for your father-in-law eventually and we'll talk about it then.' "

Knowing that the University of Pennsylvania scientists are interested in finding the cause of Alzheimer's disease, Linda has repeatedly offered some of her own pet theories—again, to no response. "I think it's the chemicals in the fertilizer on the farm," she says, a little embarrassed at her own temerity. "One of the articles I read—and I don't know my chemistry at all—mentioned something about a chemical compound, and I mentioned it to Lennie at the time I was reading it. He said, 'Well, that was always a common ingredient in fertilizers years ago.' I keep thinking, maybe they all lived on that farm for a long time and were exposed to that particular chemical."

Linda has also been looking into the genetic background of the Scott family, and she believes Mom Scott, not Pop Scott, may be the missing link. "In one item that came from the Alzheimer's Disease Society," she says, "it said one of the things they were researching was the similarity between Alzheimer's disease and Parkinson's disease, and that in the very, very distant future they may be able to treat Alzheimer's in much the same way that they treat

Parkinson's, with this L-dopa. So right away, I said to Mom, 'Hey, wait a minute. We've been talking about Grandpop having it and passing it down to Dad; but Grandmom has had Parkinson's disease for years.' Maybe it's because of the combination of the two together that there are so many children in this family that we think are affected. Maybe that's why there's a stronger link here.

"For a short period of time, we also thought that Grandpop and Grandmom were first cousins. But we talked about the family tree with people in the family, and from what we can read from the family tree they're not first cousins, but they *are* second cousins."

Linda and Leonard are incessantly climbing that family tree, looking for clues about their own futures. So far, they count Stanley, his father, his grandfather, and perhaps as many as two more sisters and a brother all afflicted with Alzheimer's disease. One of Stanley's sisters, Joan, was forced to quit her waitressing job at the age of forty-eight because of memory lapses. The doctors at the University of Pennsylvania have tested Joan, Linda says, and seem to think she shows early signs of Alzheimer's disease. Anna, another sister, moved to Florida when her forgetfulness became obvious, and the stories drifting North are that she is in bad shape. By the age of fifty, her forgetfulness was so debilitating that her husband left her. Today, Anna is fifty-two, and she has gotten lost in the neighborhood so often that her son is thinking about putting her into a nursing home.

Of Stanley's six brothers and sisters who still live nearby, only two so far have taken up Bertha's suggestion to go to the University of Pennsylvania to be tested themselves for signs of Alzheimer's disease: Aunt Joan, whose report was equivocal, and Uncle John, who received a clean bill of health. The other siblings flatly refuse to cooperate in the testing. "Uncle Fred, well, you might as well forget him," says Leonard. "He is so stubborn and so set in his ways. He lives by the clock: at quarter after seven he does this, at seven-thirty he does that; eight o'clock on Thursday night he goes to the food store and does his shopping; Saturday night he goes out but he's home by twelve. That's it. His life is planned, and to try to disrupt that—I think there's something wrong there. He was never like that before. He was always fairly easygoing. But now, man, his life is just like a book. Every day's the same." Could his regimentation be a sign that the disease process has already started? "It looks like it to me."

Linda is angry at the aunts and uncles who will not cooperate in the University of Pennsylvania program—primarily, she says, because their refusal is an affront to Bertha. "But I also feel we owe something to their children, to the cousins. The more help everybody gives, there might not be any answers for these generations, but eventually there'll be an answer for somebody. . . . I think you have an obligation to other people. And I'm going to feel guilty someday, if I'm still living and I watch those cousins face that kind of tragedy simply because no one was willing to stir up trouble and shake them by the shoulder and say, 'Hey, look, this could be happening to your mother and it could happen to you. Do something.' "

Linda is most worried about the futures of her own daughters, who are now eight and eleven and are already asking whether they will develop the same "problem" that Pop-Pop has. "If it continues as strongly as it seems to be in this family," she says, "I think my children deserve an explanation and they have to make the choice about whether to have children of their own. I don't think I would have the right to say to them 'do' or 'don't' have children. But I sit here and think I may never be able to have grandchildren. That bothers me. And I'm even more bothered thinking of my children having to make decisions about prospective husbands. They will have to tell them, 'I may carry this.' Even if they agree not to have children, to a certain extent I think they owe it to their husbands to tell them, 'You may have to take care of me.' They're going to have to choose husbands far more wisely than they would not knowing this."

"You got stuck with a winner, didn't you, kid?" says Leonard.

"Who knows? I keep telling Lennie I'll be arthritic before anything happens to him. You don't know that when you marry somebody; there are no guarantees. And Alzheimer's disease is not something that happens where you lose a child immediately. My girls will have to face the fact that maybe it's going to happen to their child in fifty years, and maybe not."

Before he drove a truck, Leonard ran his own plumbing business. Before that, he worked with his father for a construction company. Even then, before his illness, Stanley was impossible on the job. "Dad was like a wild man. He ran constantly all day long, chasing people, pushing them out of his way: 'You can't do it, let me in there.' And he got worse and worse. If you stopped for a coffee break, man, that was terrible."

Now, Leonard keeps thinking that if only his father were a calmer, more orderly man, his disease would not be so debilitating. "If he would just slow down and calm himself," he muses. "He's like a bull in a china shop. Before, when he could think and reason and it came to him, it didn't make too much difference—though he has smashed a couple of guys' hands and things like that because he got in too much of a hurry. You just couldn't work fast enough to make him happy. If you weren't running, you weren't working."

If he were to get Alzheimer's disease, Leonard says, his reaction to the frustration of forgetting would, he hopes, be different from Stanley's. "If I were in Dad's position, since I'm slower anyway, maybe I would take my time and try to reason things out a little better. But who knows? Maybe you just lose that capacity. Maybe you can't even think that way, maybe you can't rationalize. I think I would take my time a little more and maybe try to do things even though I couldn't do them." Leonard already uses a notebook to jot down driving directions after he hauls his load to a new location. "You can't remember four or five places a week. How are you going to remember that? Some guys can; I can't."

Leonard says if he found himself forgetting names, the way his father did in the first stages of his illness, he would not be too worried about his forgetfulness being an early sign of Alzheimer's disease. "I've always had a problem remembering people's names. I can remember the names of all the terminal managers, because I have to remember their names; you can't call somebody on the phone and say, 'Hey, you.' But drivers—there must be four or five hundred drivers, and I might see a guy this week and never see him again for two or three months. And two or three months from now, I'll know the guy, but what the heck's his name? But a lot of those people remember *my* name. Every once in a while, it makes me think, Now, how come they can remember my name and I can't remember theirs?"

Leonard may look exactly like Stanley, but he does not feel as though he knows him very well. "Dad doesn't talk," he says. "He never did. I don't remember ever actually discussing anything with him. Even at the dinner table when we were kids, we never talked about anything. He was always in too much of a rush. He's been in a rush forever." Still, Stanley now has chosen Leonard as the favorite son—"the only one that doesn't holler at him, the only one that doesn't give him a hard time, the only one that doesn't pick on him," is how Bertha tells it. And Stanley has tried, after a lifetime of silence, to begin opening up to Leonard.

"He's talked to me a couple of times sitting out there on the bench under the tree," Leonard says. "He's said, you know, he'll tell you that he knows he can't remember. He always brings it up; I haven't yet. But what can you tell him? There's nothing I can do to help him except try to be a friend to him. I don't have any answers. What do you say?"

Life with Father: Steven and Jane

"Sometimes I get mad at him; I forget that he's sick," says Steven Scott, who, as Stanley's business partner, bears the brunt these days of Stanley's temper, forgetfulness, and rage. "The doctors want him to stay active, they want him to stay working at the yard. They've told me, 'He has to stay active or he'll go too fast.' But nobody looks at my side, what it's costing to have him there. Still, I guess we don't have much choice in the matter."

Steve resembles Bertha, not Stanley, but his temper is said to be as hot as his father's. Now, talking about Stanley's problem and the way it disrupts business, he mumbles and swallows his words. He does not want to look as though he is complaining—but neither does he want his junkyard run into the ground.

"It's getting so it costs me more to keep him up there than I pay him for his salary. It costs me $300 or $400 a week for some of the stuff he does sometimes. One day he got mad and punched out the windows in a car—I had paid $500 for that car. It had a nice front assembly on it that was worth $500, and he ruined it. It was hit pretty bad in the back so it wouldn't slide off the truck, so he got mad at it and rammed it with the forklift. There goes $500 right out the window.

"I've got to spend too much time watching him. There's not much he can do. He shouldn't even be delivering parts alone, I guess. He has his pet things that he likes to do, like check the transmission fluid in the truck. Every time he uses the truck he's got to put transmission fluid in it, even if it overflows. He just doesn't understand what he's doing a lot of the time."

Even the simple jobs are falling out of Stanley's reach. "I asked him to get the mail the other day," Steve says, "and he just looked at me, like, Where do you get the mail? I said, 'What's the matter?' and he said, 'I've never gotten the mail.' He goes down almost every day to get the mail."

Steve thought a good task for his father would be to put drums and rotors from junked cars into the bins in the supply room. But it wasn't. "The drums are numbered and the bin is numbered," Steve says. "He can't even put a 1452 drum in a 1452 bin. He just can't even read the four numbers and get the four numbers together. So when you sell a 1452 rotor that's on the inventory, you go out there and it's not in the right spot, and you don't know where it's at. You can't even have him do that."

The crane that Stanley has operated his whole adult life has become almost a lethal weapon in Stanley's confused hands. "One day he had the crane hooked up to the motor of a car, and he was trying to get the motor out [to prepare the car for the scrap heap]," says Steve. "The motor was stuck; it wouldn't come out. He's got the car all the way up in the air just held by the motor, so if the motor does come out the car's coming down. And he's standing underneath it, prying the motor out with a crowbar. I told him to get out from underneath there, and he almost had a heart attack: 'Don't you think I know what I'm doing?' I said, 'Yeah, you're trying to kill yourself, that's what you're doing.' I don't think he realized what would happen when he was under there. I pulled him out and tried to explain to him but all he'd say was 'Don't you think I know what I'm doing?' "

Playing nursemaid to his father is trying Steve's patience, which is already in limited supply. Stanley has become a menace around the yard. He will take a torch to a car to remove its motor, forgetting first to empty its gasoline tank. He will go to a car lot and load brand-new cars onto the truck and haul them back to the junkyard, instead of taking the old cars ready for the trash heap. "It's tough to sit there and watch him not know how to do something," says his son, "or take a sledgehammer to open a trunk. He'll work himself to death—he works so hard, and he does nothing. It really gets you to see him sit there not knowing that he could just reach in the car and take the key out to open the trunk. He won't think to look—or, if he looks and it's not in there, he won't think to just take the torch and cut the lock out. He'll beat it to death instead and work up a sweat and use up so much energy—and do nothing. He goes home at night and he's completely worn out, but at the end of the day he hasn't done an hour's worth of work."

The customers do not seem to know what to make of Stanley. "Ever since we started building the crusher, he's just been unbearable," Steve says. "A customer comes in and asks what it is, and he'll rant and rave about it. The customer doesn't want to hear that. Even if it's a woman customer, he'll cuss and swear about that crusher. They look at you like, What's going on here?

159

"For a while he was on a current events kick. People would come into the yard and he would start talking about things he read in the paper—but he'd have it all messed up. I don't know what the people thought. There he was, talking and talking like he was an expert on everything, but he just had it all wrong. Some people would try to correct him, and he would argue with them. Some people, especially the women, would just back away. When he was talking like that, it was like they were afraid of him."

Steve knows that if he booted his father out of the business, he would be sentencing him to an even emptier life. But he does not know if there are any jobs left that Stanley can handle. Steve turned down an offer of $3,000 for the crane—"I couldn't sell that crane; it's Dad's baby"—even though the machine will only be taking up space once the crusher is in operation. "I keep thinking maybe I can let it sit in a corner of the yard and let Dad play with it." Steve will soon have to force his father to stop making delivery runs in the company truck—he is thinking of buying a new tractor-trailer that Stanley will not know how to drive—and may even decide that operating the crusher, a simple job that entails pressing three levers, is beyond him. "I've tried to tell him that he'll be able to run the crusher. But I'm at the point where I don't know if I want him to run it because he might break it just to prove it's no good. I don't want to put $5,000 into something just to have him beat it to death." and Stanley is not above sabotaging the machine, says Steve, to prove that Steve had wasted their money by building the crusher. "He keeps saying that crane can run for another five years," Steve says. "But he's the only one that can run that crane, and you can't have a piece of equipment that nobody can run."

Steve's wife, Jane, is a quiet woman with the same round face and dark coloring of her husband. She works in a local factory on the night shift, cares for her two little boys during the day, and rarely manages to get in more than a few hours' worth of sleep at a time. Her approach to the notion that Alzheimer's disease runs in the Scott family is matter-of-fact; she plans no grand talks for her sons in explaining about inheritance patterns and the wisdom of having children of their own. "They're going to be living it. They're going to see it. God forbid if somebody else gets it that's closer to them even than Pop-Pop, they're going to be even more aware of it."

Steve says he cannot plan for that time, fifteen or twenty years from now. "Fifteen years is too far away. I got too much to do now to worry about fifteen years from now. I'm not going to worry about it until the time comes." His wife disagrees. "You can't just shut it out of your mind and say if it happens in fifteen years I'm going to start worrying about it then," Jane says.

"I'm not shutting it out of my mind," says Steve, his voice rising. "I'm just not going to get involved in worrying about it right now."

"Yes, but there are things you can do to plan accordingly . . ."

"You can't plan nothing on that."

"You can. Maybe you can live a little different, and think a little different. Sometimes, as rough as it is now, you think if that's going to come, too, then what years are going to come when we can enjoy each other, when things aren't going to be as hard? Maybe when those years finally come, it's going to be even worse."

Perhaps the hardest part for Steve about having his father at the junkyard every day is that he is not allowed the luxury of putting the future out of his mind for a while. He does not want to think about what his own later years might be like, "but it's getting tough not to. I don't know if I could put up with it, if I ever get like that. I don't want to be around. You're actually useless. You can't do anything." He can understand, far more than can his brother or his mother, that Stanley might really mean it when he threatens to kill himself. "He has enough sense about him to know that he can't do anything, and then what's the sense of being around? You're not accomplishing anything, you have no usefulness anymore. You're putting a burden on everybody. I think he's still smart enough to realize that."

The Professional Opinion

"Stanley's in bad shape," says Jack Friedman, who was for a time the Scotts' family therapist from Ardmore, Pennsylvania. "He's not that aware of what's going on around him. But I don't think he's hurting as much as his actions would indicate. I think he's got less inhibition about showing certain kinds of feelings—he is more prone to be irritated, more prone to have a temper tantrum, more prone to get angry, more prone to cry. But I'm not sure that when he does these things he feels them any more [than other people do]; in fact, my guess is that when he does these things he probably makes the response but feels it less. When the brain begins to go, especially the cerebral cortex as in Alzheimer's disease, you get massive behavioral shifts. Dogs, for example, who have been experimentally decorticated bare their teeth and growl. But if you go up to the dogs and pet them, you'll find they're perfectly docile."

Friedman specializes in the study of family "time bombs"—legacies which some individuals expect to inherit by a certain date, such as an early death by heart attack, and which color their entire lives. Alzheimer's disease, especially in the Scott family, is such a "time bomb." "Events which happen randomly in this particular family cannot be considered random," Friedman says. "If I get up and go across the room and then forget what I'm going for, it doesn't bother me. If I leave the house and I forget my keys, or if I have an appointment and I happen to miss it, I'll say something like 'Well, I have too much on my mind.' If Leonard does that, immediately it becomes suspect and it starts panicking him."

If acknowledged early enough, the "time bomb" can sometimes be defused. "Alzheimer's disease is the kind of event, or life situation, which can enrich a life, make it deeper and more meaningful, as well as destroy it. It has the potential to do both. It can make the family come to terms with what life is all about. Whether they spend their money now and live it up, or postpone some of their gratification for retirement age, is not the real relevant issue. The relevant issue is that when they're confronted with this question now, they have to go dig into themselves and determine what values they're going to live by, what things are important to them. If their relationship is important, then it should get stronger and they should get closer and they should be able to share more."

Friedman's real patient, he says, is not Stanley, for whom he and other doctors believe they can do very little. The real patient is the rest of the Scott family: Bertha, Leonard and Linda, Steve and Jane, and even those of Stanley's brothers and sisters who are willing to take part. His counseling, Friedman hopes, can build a stronger family network, which may coincidentally help Stanley cope for a longer period of time. A supportive spouse or family probably will not retard the organic disease, he says, "but if there's a good deal of love and caring you can tolerate a person a lot longer and can keep the system going without having to resort to some kind of convalescent or nursing home."

Weighing Stanley's need for continued activity against Steve's need for independence, tranquillity, and a business that functions, Friedman seems to come down in favor of keeping Stanley at the junkyard for as long as possible: "We know certain things about this kind of organic problem. We know that if you get isolated and withdrawn, the process speeds up. It's as though the ego needs a situation that is a challenging one in order to continue to function.

"Stanley has always been a domineering father. Steve is trying to be independent and to run the business, and Stanley is very confused about who the business belongs to. I think they're in partnership financially, so [the junkyard] is not simply Steve's, even though Steve feels as though it is up to him to run it. I don't think the problems here are that much different from those in other families where the father and son are in business and the father feels pushed aside with the son taking over."

Many of the family's problems now, says Friedman, are the result not of Alzheimer's disease itself but of long-established family patterns. "This kind of illness magnifies the existing personality. Stanley has always been stubborn. Stanley has always had temper tantrums. Stanley, when he didn't get his way, has always chewed other people out. He's always put his kids down if they disagreed with him; he's always intimidated Bertha. That's nothing new. All he's doing is doing it on a less rational basis."

Stanley's neurologist, Howard Hurtig of the University of Pennsylvania medical center, has a slightly different view: To Hurtig, many of Stanley's current problems are the direct result of the disease process itself. Violence is often a part of the clinical picture of Alzheimer's disease, even in the most even-tempered of patients, "because the brain is involved. When the brain deteriorates, anything can happen. The temporal lobe of the brain [in which the largest proportion of neuritic plaques and neurofibrillary tangles are found] is intimately related to the emotional center of the brain, the so-called limbic system." And unlike Friedman, who thinks Stanley's temper tantrums are superficial evidences of what is in fact a shallow range of emotion, Hurtig believes the "fits" are probably as difficult for Stanley to go through as they are for the family to witness. "He may have certain built-in protection by virtue of his memory disorder, by not being able to remember how bad things are or how good he used to be," Hurtig says, but while Stanley is crying, he is feeling pain.

The neurologist does not share his patient's enthusiasm about lecithin. "I don't expect him to get much better on lecithin," he admits. "The only reason we give it to him is that there is a theoretical reason why lecithin might work, and some people have tried it in patients with Alzheimer's disease. The results have not been clear-cut, so until we have some better answers I think it's reasonable to go ahead and try it on people. It's a harmless drug."

Nor does Hurtig share the Scott family's conviction that they may all be doomed to inherit Alzheimer's disease. "There's no specific genetic pattern, unlike something like Huntington's disease, where you know what the probable risk is of getting it. In Alzheimer's it's not at all like that and, in fact, most people who have it do not have other affected family members." Scientists' best information, he says, is that only about 10 to 15 percent of the families in which Alzheimer's disease is found will have more than one family member affected, "but it's not as though they're all brothers and sisters; you might instead have a cousin or an uncle or an aunt affected."

To the idea that the "pre-senile" form of dementia—the kind that Stanley has—is a different disease from "senile dementia," Hurtig offers a sharp, "Baloney." To the notion that the familial and non-familial forms of Alzheimer's disease are different, he is somewhat less committal. "But all of these ideas are born out of ignorance," he says, "and I think we will find in time that Alzheimer's disease is a continuum as part of the aging process, and something happens in some people to trigger it off early. That's probably a genetic factor."

Hurtig participated in a three-year, multi-university project, funded by the NIA, designed to uncover the role of genetics, environment, and other factors in the development of Alzheimer's disease. To do so, Hurtig and his co-workers searched for common threads in the life stories of some 100 persons with Alzheimer's disease—threads that might not appear in the stories of the age-matched control subjects who were studied at the same time. Stanley Scott volunteered to be one of the 100 Alzheimer's disease subjects. His sister, Joan, was also in the study.

How strong is the genetic link to Alzheimer's disease in the Scott family? "It is less real than we thought originally," Hurtig points out. "When they first came in here, they told me that everybody had Alzheimer's disease, and then we started getting family members to come in. One brother clearly did not have it. Joan Maynes, Stanley's sister, probably does have it, but her case is not that easy to figure out either. If you accept her as a case, that's just two out of ten"—Stanley and Joan out of the original ten siblings. But what about Anna, supposedly fast losing her mind down in Florida? "That's the thing you have to be very careful about," Hurtig says. "People often start developing an illness after it's been identified in the family. That's the trouble with doing genetic research."

The trouble is especially aggravated in genetic research into a disease like Alzheimer's, which is so difficult to diagnose with certainty. When Scott family members are called to the University of Pennsylvania for testing, they go through such examinations as a spinal tap, an electroencephalogram, and a CT scan, but these physical tests are done only to rule out other possible causes of mental problems. The most helpful tests in the diagnosis of Alzheimer's are psychological measures of memory and orientation. "In other tests, such as the CT scan, there's too much variability to be of much help," says Hurtig. "For example, Stanley Scott's CT scan is fairly normal, yet he's got a profound memory disturbance. But many people with mild dementia can have fairly severely abnormal CT scans. We're not really sure what it means."

The plaques and tangles, which are the only sure signs of Alzheimer's disease, can only be observed, short of autopsy, after a brain biopsy. This involves removing a piece of the brain itself through a hole drilled in the skull. "It would be major surgery in Alzheimer's disease because the disease concentrates in the inner part of the brain, so in order to get at the part that is most affected, you would have to go deep into the brain. It's not worth it, because if you've excluded most of the other possible diagnoses, then you're most likely left with Alzheimer's disease. There are very few other diseases that behave like that."

The prevailing theory about the genetics of Alzheimer's disease, Hurtig says, is that it is a "polygenetic illness"—that is, the tendency to develop Alzheimer's, like the tendency to develop Parkinson's disease, lupus erythematosis, and many other diseases, is probably carried on several genes. "There is this sort of potential for having it, and then if something comes along in the environment that triggers it, it will precipitate the disease." An alternative theory, and one to which Hurtig himself does not subscribe, is that the tendency for Alzheimer's disease is carried on only one gene—as it is in illnesses such as Huntington's and Tay-Sachs, which follow a predictable genetic pattern—and that the gene has "variable penetrance, which means there is a single gene that is penetrating some people and not others. Penetrance is thought to be determined by individual host factors. So if someone is strong and resistant, then maybe the disease would not show up, or would show up very late in life." To Hurtig's way of thinking, the idea of a single gene with variable penetrance as a cause of Alzheimer's is only a different, and less plausible, way of describing a disease of polygenetic origin triggered by environmental factors.

Hurtig's theories cannot help him predict what will happen to Stanley Scott—or to his children and grandchildren. "Alzheimer's disease is clearly a progessive disease," he says. "The natural history of it is not predictable, even though the outcome is predictable. Many people will stand still for a long time and then may suddenly get worse. I had a patient once with this disease who was slowly getting worse and then within a month she had died. She had rapidly deteriorated for no apparent reason. She became vegetative, couldn't function at all, went into a nursing home, and died."

Part of "the mythology, the black magic" surrounding Alzheimer's disease is the belief that if you keep pushing yourself, keep trying to remember, you will decline less rapidly. Hurtig doubts that such factors have any bearing on the progression of the illness itself. But as far as Stanley Scott keeping active—holding on to his job as long as he can, maintaining such privileges as driving a car—Hurtig thinks it will help the family, and probably Stanley, to cope with his progressive losses if he has something diverting to do. "If he's working, my feeling about Stanley, not knowing him terribly well, is that he has a better self-image if he's able to stay occupied. That's true of all of us; if you sit around and do nothing, you shrivel up."

As for Leonard and Steven, Hurtig is not even laying odds. Though both sons would gladly submit to some baseline psychological or physiological testing to see whether they seem likely to develop Alzheimer's disease, Hurtig says he would not offer such tests even if there were any to give. "The genetic pattern is so unpredictable that you're really putting a terrible stigma on someone by even subjecting him to the tests. What if you found an abnormality? How would you interpret that? What if they planned their lives along a certain pathway and then found out at the end of that that the test had been wrong?"

Hurtig recalls a seminar on genetic screening he attended in which the panel leader, to demonstrate our own tendency to shun predictions, distributed sealed envelopes to members of the audience. "In each of these envelopes," he said, "is the date of your own death. When I count to three, you may open them. One, two, three." No one opened the envelope that supposedly foretold his future.

"You always want to hope that you're going to escape the fate of your family," Hurtig explains. And by encouraging the younger Scotts to live their lives as normally as they can, he is giving them room for that hope.

Epilogue

Six years have passed since these conversations with the Scotts took place. According to Howard Hurtig, now chairman of the Department of Neurology at the Graduate Hospital of the University of Pennsylvania, Stanley is just about the same as he was six years ago. "His condition has progressed some—he can't do much for himself—and his family sees him as being much worse than he was a few years ago," Hurtig says. "But in superficial conversation he seems fine, or at least as fine as he seemed when I first knew him, and on the fairly simple tests that I give him in my office I haven't seen much change."

Hurtig says the Scotts have stopped Stanley from driving the car—it was just too dangerous—and have stopped him from working at the junkyard. Stanley takes Haldol, a tranquilizer, to control his outbursts of temper, and he still lives at home with Bertha. As for the federal study Hurtig was involved in in which Stanley and his sister participated, not much was revealed about the possible precursors of Alzheimer's disease. "There did seem to be more thyroid problems among the patients with Alzheimer's disease, but we don't know what that means," Hurtig says. "And we confirmed the findings that were made by several other groups of the higher prevalence of Down's syndrome in Alzheimer's families."

Less than three years after Linda Scott talked about her family's future, she died suddenly of a brain aneurysm. Leonard and his two daughters now live on a horse farm not far from the house Leonard had built. Theresa Browne, a woman who went to high school with Leonard and Linda and who gave riding lessons to their older daughter, lives with them on the farm. "Everyone seems to have come through the worst of their hard times." Theresa says. But the clock is still ticking, and Stanley Scott's sons are now less than ten years away from the age at which their father developed Alzheimer's disease. The eerily apt sentiment that Linda had expressed—that when it comes to the future, "there are no guarantees"—means that the Scotts' story is still being told.

7

Senility "Cures": The Far Out and the Possible

When doctors can offer patients no hope, patients often seek hope in other quarters. That's what has been happening in the case of Alzheimer's disease and, to a lesser extent, in the cases of people suffering the other, less severe mental changes of old age. Like the diagnosis of cancer, which has sent thousands to the spas and clinics that promise cures through laetrile, vitamins, or mineral baths, the diagnosis of dementia stirs up the kinds of fears and uncertainties that make people search desperately for something, anything, that offers added years of a fuller, easier life. Many physicians are hesitant to stop their patients with Alzheimer's disease from searching for nostrums and cures that harm nothing but the pocketbook. What price tag can be placed on hope?

The agony behind the search for a fountain of youth has been with us for generations. But for the first time, it seems, the efforts are directed toward ways to rejuvenate the mind housed within a still-functioning body—rather than, as it was in years past, to rejuvenate the body housing a still-functioning mind. Years ago, people aged physically with startling quickness (James Whistler's mother, that archetype of old age, was only forty-four years old when she sat for her famous portrait in 1872). Few survived long enough to lose their mental sharpness; the body decayed while the mind stayed young. The Irish poet William Butler Yeats, one of a select group of people who submitted to "monkey gland" implantation earlier in this century to restore his physical prowess, maintained an awesome acuity that made the state of his aged body all the more loathsome to him. As he lamented in 1927, when he was sixty-two years old:

> What shall I do with this absurdity—
> O heart, O troubled heart—this caricature,
> Decrepit age that has been tied to me
> As to a dog's tail?
>   Never had I more
> Excited, passionate, fantastical
> Imagination, nor an ear and eye
> That more expected the impossible—

Today, doctors are far more able to correct the "caricature," the physical changes of old age, than they are to reignite the "fantastical imagination" that Yeats maintained long after his body had withered. For 2 to 3 million Americans with Alzheimer's disease, this failure of modern medicine sentences them to a life in which their bodies, still healthy, house ever-sicker, ever-emptier brains.

So the race is on to find ways to circumvent the sentence of death-in-life that Alzheimer's disease can mean. And, trailing right behind, millions more Americans are rushing toward an elusive remedy for aging itself, including the forgetfulness and confusion that often accompany aging. Leading the pack are proponents of food and dietary supplements, who offer nostrums that can be purchased in health food stores or pharmacies without a physician's okay. Moving with more deliberation are the scientists conducting clinical trials on a wide range of drugs and techniques that offer some hope of alleviating the symptoms of Alzheimer's disease, as well as some of the milder mental changes of age. And progressing most cautiously of all are the basic scientists, hoping against hope that a cause for the disease—slow virus, genetics, metal toxicity, or some combination—will be found that implies not a stopgap treatment, but a cure.

In this chapter, we will describe some of the methods that have been tried to minimize the symptoms of Alzheimer's disease and the milder mental symptoms of very old age. None of them is yet part of standard medical treatment for Alzheimer's disease, because none has yet been proved either safe or effective. They are offered here only as a taste of things to come—and as proof of the fervor with which people, laymen and scientists alike, are searching still for a fountain of youth.

The Self-Help Route

Perhaps the most exciting discovery in the neurosciences during the last decade was the finding that we are what we eat. To a greater extent than was ever thought possible, the environment of the brain was found to be alterable on a daily or perhaps even an hourly basis, depending on what we had for lunch or dinner. At the same time, dietary approaches to mental problems gained popularity, such as the controversial Feingold additive-free diet for hyperactive children. Articles and books touting new kinds of "mind foods" began to appear, urging people to rush to the neighborhood health food store for packages of nutrients, vitamins, and supplements likely to increase the amount of "good" neurotransmitters or proteins in the brain. Persons with Alzheimer's disease, and elderly persons troubled by forgetfulness, probably were among the first to heed the call. Many of the remedies offered—choline and lecithin, vitamin E, nicotinic acid, ribonucleic acid (RNA)—specifically promised improvements in memory, as did the purported youth drug, available in this country only in Nevada, known as Gerovital H-3.

The rationale for each of these therapies differs. In the cases of choline or lecithin and RNA, the thought is that replacement of substances missing in the aged brain, and missing to an even greater extent in the brains of Alzheimer's patients, would restore the brain to full functioning. In the case of vitamin E, the thought is that a destructive brain process—bombardment by molecules known as free radicals—can be inhibited. Nicotinic acid, also called niacin or vitamin B_3, is thought to correct the nutritional deficiency presumed to underlie senile behavior. And Gerovital H-3, its proponents say, seems capable of inhibiting the action of one of the "bad" neurotransmitters found in great quantities in the older brain.

Although the reasoning in each case makes logical sense —trying to replace what has been lost, or to reverse biological activities that seem destructive—results with each of these remedies have so far been disappointing. But some doctors are prescribing dietary supplements to their patients with Alzheimer's disease in the hope that scientific logic will outweigh experimental disappointment. To them, some therapy is better than no therapy.

THE SELF-HELP ROUTE, I: CHOLINE AND LECITHIN

The fuss began in 1974, when David Drachman, a neurologist then at Northwestern University, administered a drug called scopolamine to a group of normal, healthy college students. The students began to act "senile." While maintaining their verbal skills and their immediate memory, the students revealed impairment of memory storage and general cognitive functioning, and the electroencephalogram patterns, like the EEGs of patients with Alzheimer's disease, showed more slow waves, particularly over the temporal lobes of the brain. The findings were significant because of the known action of scopolamine: it blocks the movement of the neurotransmitter acetylcholine in the brain.

Acetylcholine is part of the cholinergic system of neurotransmitters, and scientists in the late 1970s were beginning to think the cholinergic system played a crucial role in memory formation. They were learning, too, that the balance of the neurotransmitter could be modified by what we eat and what drugs we take. John Fernstrom and Richard Wurtman of the Massachusetts Institute of Technology were among the first to report that the feeding of substances containing choline, which is necessary for the synthesis of acetylocholine, increased the amount of transmitter in a crucial part of the brain: the hippocampus.

At about the time this choline connection was discovered, Peter Davies, a British scientist now at New York's Albert Einstein Medical College, forged another link in the experimental chain. He found that the amount of enzyme needed to turn choline into acetylcholine was a remarkable 91 percent lower in Alzheimer's disease patients than in normal aged individuals. What would happen, scientists then began to wonder, if we simply put back the missing acetylcholine? Drachman had done it in his experiments with healthy college students, whose acetylcholine levels had been artifically reduced with drugs. Their mental functioning had been restored when they were given choline directly in order to counteract the effects of the scopolamine; their acetylcholine levels thus returned to normal. Could the same thing be done with elderly people, especially those suffering from Alzheimer's disease?

At New York University, Steven Ferris, Samuel Gershon, and Gregory Sathananthan administered a drug called Deanol to fourteen elderly patients with mild to moderate impairment of mental functioning. Deanol is thought to increase the level of acetylcholine in the brain. After four weeks of taking the drug three times a day, ten of the patients showed some improvement and four of the patients showed none. But the improvement was in behavioral rather than mental symptoms: Deanol seemed to relieve depression, irritability, and anxiety, but did little to improve the subjects' performance on tests of memory and other cognitive functions.

The NYU group also tried to raise the acetylcholine level in the brain through the administration of choline chloride, a form of choline. On a graduated dosage schedule of from 12 to 20 grams of choline chloride per day, depending on the individual's tolerance, the subjects showed no improvement after taking the drug for a total of four weeks. This test with choline chloride was confirmed in numerous other studies around the country in the late 1970s. In one, seven patients with advanced cases of Alzheimer's disease showed no improvement after four weeks of choline chloride treatment of up to 10 grams per day; in another, eight normal elderly subjects taking 16 grams of choline chloride every day for a week similarly showed no improvement in memory storage, retrieval, mood, or social functioning. Scientists have a theory about why choline replacement

176

therapy seems to defy the apparent logic that says more acetylcholine should lead to better memory; very old people with memory problems, or individuals with Alzheimer's disease, might have lost more than the enzymes and compounds needed to manufacture acetylcholine. They might somehow have lost the very ability to turn choline into acetylcholine even if all the raw ingredients are present. In addition, Peter Davies has found that at least one other neurotransmitter, somatostatin, also is decreased in persons with Alzheimer's disease. For treatment with choline or lecithin to work, he says, the somatostatin transmitter system may have to be beefed up as well.

In 1984 scientists at the Dartmouth-Hitchcock Medical Center in New Hampshire reported some success with a form of acetylcholine called bethanechol. But this was not just a dietary technique; this involved delivering the acetylcholine directly into the ventricles of the brain. The researchers, led by Dr. Robert Harbaugh, implanted a catheter into the brain through a hole in the skull, and connected the catheter to a small infusion pump implanted under the skin of the abdomen. Harbaugh's preliminary work involved only four patients, but the results were encouraging. According to family members' reports, the patients showed improvement in social activity, personal hygiene, conversational abilities, and even such skills as reading. More research is needed, however, before the technique goes beyond the purely experimental.

The allure of a dietary component to stimulate brain activity is irresistible. Choline is readily available through such sources as eggs, organ meats, and fish or, even more readily, in the form of lecithin, a component found in soybeans, yeast, and liver. Lecithin is also used as an emulsifier in cake mixes, chocolates, gelatin mixes, gravies, salad dressing, and other prepared foods, and is sold in individual packets in health food stores. Could a meal of a large omelet

177

or an extra three ounces a day of lecithin render an otherwise forgetful old man ready for a winning game of chess?

Scientists are hesitant to state unequivocally that a diet high in choline or lecithin will improve the mental prowess of the aged — or, for that matter, of the young. They advise against a rush to the local health food store, where lecithin has been selling for years. The damage, some point out, could be more than a financial one: the lecithin on the market is only 20 percent active lecithin, and the remaining 80 percent is unanalyzed. For an individual to ingest the 100 grams of lecithin thought of as a sufficient daily dose, he would have to ingest an extra 700 calories, too. In addition, choline has been shown to exhibit what scientists call a biphasic effect, meaning that the wrong amount of the substance — either too much *or* too little — could lead to an actual decline in intellectual performance. What's more, choline is metabolized by certain intestinal bacteria in such a way that it often causes people taking large doses to give off an unpleasant, fishy odor.

THE SELF-HELP ROUTE, II: VITAMIN E

The advertisements for vitamin E call it the anti-aging vitamin. Sold in soft capsules encasing a jelly-like, squishy pill, vitamin E is said to fight wrinkles, hair loss, and sagging skin. The claims made are so dramatic — and the presence of vitamin E supplements in certain cosmetic creams is so heralded — that many people are wary of the vitamin's ability to do anything but make its promoters richer. But at least one medical scientist believes that vitamin E is a good method for fighting senile dementia.

Denham Harman, a chemist at the University of Nebraska, first proposed his "free radical theory of aging" in 1966. Free radicals are highly unstable pieces of molecules that are on the prowl for other molecules to link up with. Harman believes that the hookup of free radicals with other molecules underlies the basic process of cellular aging, in the brain and in other parts of the body. Among the damage done by the intruding free radicals, which attach to molecule segments in ways that prevent the affected molecule from performing its job, is the formation of amyloid in various organs. Amyloid, as we have seen, is a major constituent of the neuritic plaques found to some extent in the brains of all old people and to a far greater extent in persons with Alzheimer's disease. And vitamin E, Harman says, can retard this process of free radical formation and amyloid production through its anti-oxidant properties. By reducing the amount of available oxygen in the cells, the theory goes, vitamin E limits the production of free radicals (which need oxygen for their generation), and thus prevents the mischief they may do.

THE SELF-HELP ROUTE, III: NICOTINIC ACID

The Canadian physician A. Hoffer says he was an unwilling convert to the powers of nicotinic acid. In 1954 he offered his mother megadoses of the substance, also known as niacin or vitamin B_3, because she obviously was deteriorating rapidly. At age sixty-seven, her memory and her vision were failing, she had become nervous, depressed, weak, and easily fatigued, bothered as well by severe arthritis in both hands. Nicotinic acid, Hoffer knew, was believed to increase the rate of tissue repair and reduce the amount of cholesterol in the blood, but he offered the vitamin "more or less as a placebo. . . . It was relatively less toxic than is senility itself."

The doctor was "amazed" to see an almost total recovery in his mother within six weeks. When she was eighty-five years old, and had been taking 3 grams of nicotinic acid every day for eighteen years, Hoffer reported triumphantly to a conference at the Huxley Institute for Biosocial Research in New York that "she is physically weaker, does not hear as well, but is mentally well. . . . I have not seen any evidence of toxicity, and there has been no progression of the mental senility which was so apparent eighteen years ago." After witnessing the improvement in his mother and in others taking nicotinic acid — notably survivors of Japanese prisoner-of-war camps who, years after their release, still suffered the effects of chronic semi-starvation in the camps — Hoffer concluded that senility is "a vitamin-dependent condition which comes from many years of mild or moderate chronic vitamin deficiencies." He based his conclusion partly on the fact that the former POWs, while still in middle age, encountered many chronic problems that seemed to resemble the problems of great old age.

Hoffer insists any older person with symptoms of depression, anxiety, irritability, memory loss, confusion, and disorientation should be given 3 grams a day of nicotinic acid, which, he says, is "more specific as an anti-senility medication than any other chemical I have had much experience with. If it is started before there are irreversible anatomical or biochemical changes, the results will be much superior, but even after [the changes have] started it will probably prevent or slow down the rate of senescence [aging]." Hoffer also urges older people to "embark on a program of orthomolecular living," a kind of therapeutic approach to life that includes some radical changes in the diet — primarily the elimination of sugar. He says old people should increase their intake of high-quality protein foods, reduce their intake of saturated fats and carbohydrates, and increase the proportion of unrefined grains, rice, and cereal in relation to refined foods in the diet. Besides this orthomolecular diet, he proposes that individuals self-prescribe nutritional supplements, as needed, "in the following order: nicotinic acid, pyridoxine, ascorbic acid (vitamin C), thiamine (vitamin B_1), vitamin B_{12}, vitamin E, 1-glutamine (MSG)."

Few other physicians will venture a guess as to the anti-senility value of vitamins. Standard treatment for Alzheimer's disease in its early stages is often a daily multi-vitamin supplement, but this is as daring as most doctors get on the subject. Since nutritional research still lags far behind advances made in other areas of biomedicine, it may be years before physicians can tell their patients with any assurance what the effects of certain foods, vitamins, and minerals will be on the way they feel and the way they think.

THE SELF-HELP ROUTE, IV: RNA

RNA (ribonucleic acid) is the cousin of the genetic component DNA, which carries all of a cell's inherited information. RNA is involved in heredity, too, but it is also thought to play a role in learning and memory, through the synthesis of knowledge-specific proteins in the brain. Animal studies have shown that the amount of RNA in the brain increases after an animal has learned something new.

One example of RNA's powers is seen in an early experiment conducted by James McConnell at the University of Michigan. McConnell taught flatworms a particular trick—crawling through a maze—and then killed the worms and fed them to other flatworms who had not learned the maze. The worms who had eaten the trained worms learned the same maze significantly faster than did other untrained worms. McConnell theorized that the original worms, in learning the maze, had synthesized a particular kind of

RNA specific to that task. And the RNA carried the knowledge of that task alone; the flatworms who ate the trained worms were no quicker than any other flatworms at learning to crawl through an entirely new maze.

If RNA is indeed a learning substrate, scientists have reasoned, perhaps the introduction of extra RNA into the aged brain can help old people retain their ability to learn and to remember. D. Ewen Cameron of the Allan Memorial Institute of Psychiatry in Montreal was one of the first to test this theory in humans. Beginning in 1956, he injected RNA, as well as DNA, into twenty-three elderly patients with memory impairment, and reported favorable results in half the subjects. "The best results were obtained in patients having severe memory deficits and marked confusion. In most of these the confusion cleared up, orientation returned, and there was considerable or complete restoration of retention." He said it took four or five days to see results: if no impairment could be seen by that time, a longer trial of RNA therapy was unlikely to be of much benefit.

Scientists have been unable to replicate Cameron's optimistic findings. In 1972 Augusto Britton and his colleagues at the University of Southern California reported failure in their study of thirty-five hospitalized patients with severe memory deficits who were given RNA supplements for up to three weeks. Their results, Britton said, "must be placed with the increasing number [of studies] which indicate that memory is not improved by compounds intended to increase levels of RNA." Included under that rubric is not simply RNA itself, but such RNA-synthesizing compounds as magnesium pemoline, which has also been tried—with disappointing results—to correct memory loss in old age.

Still, many health food stores are touting the healing properties of RNA. But as Durk Pearson and Sandy Shaw write in their best-seller *Life Extension*, self-medication with RNA can be a dangerous habit for some people. Metabolism of the compound releases high levels of uric acid, which can seriously aggravate gout in people who have it and can bring on gout in people with high levels of uric acid in their systems. They suggest a uric acid test before trying RNA, and another test one month after self-administration, since "permanent damage can be done to the joints and kidneys by [uric acid] crystals." Pearson and Shaw offer a more traditional bit of advice as well. "Check the label before you buy. Yeast is about 6 percent RNA, but the plant's cell walls are so hard to digest that the body takes in very little. If a product contains less than 12 percent RNA, you are probably just buying overpriced yeast with little available nucleic acid."

THE SELF-HELP ROUTE, V: GEROVITAL H-3

A handful of spas are nestled in the Carpathian Mountains and along the Black Sea coast of Romania. The setting of each is idyllic, but the thousands of tourists who flock there each year are looking for more than rest and scenery. They are looking for youth—and they buy it in two-week "geriatric cure" vacations and batches of the preparation known as Gerovital H-3 (GH-3). If they're Americans, they return home with one-year supplies because, unless they live in the maverick state of Nevada, they won't be able to buy Gerovital H-3 at their neighborhood pharmacies. GH-3 has been banned in the United States—although sales are brisk through what the FDA calls "Mom and Pop Shops"—mail-order businesses that seek their clients through classified ads.

There's no doubt that the Romanian National Tourist Office—which sponsors several package tours of these health spas beginning at $980 off-season up to $2,060 in-season, depending on accommodations, for two-week "geriatricure tours"—has benefited from the popularity of GH-3. But what about the patients who go to Romania, some of them year after year, seeking a lost youth? What happens to them while they are there, and what are they doing for themselves when they get home and continue to self-administer the elixir that they expect to cure everything from graying hair to failing memory?

Gerovital H-3 was developed in the late 1940s by the Bucharest physician Ana Aslan. Aslan, who has an international scientific reputation, is careful in her professional claims for the drug. But her four-color portrait appears prominently in such pamphlets as the one distributed by the Carpati National Tourist Office of Bucharest, where her Geriatric Clinic is located. The brochure issues extravagant claims for Aslan's invention; GH-3 and its cousin, Aslavital, it says, can have "a favourable effect in the nervous and physical asthenia [weakness], in memory, attention and concentration capacity troubles, in the diminishing sensorial acuteness (presbyopia [diminished vision], presbycusis [loss of hearing], cataract), in neuroses and neuralgias, in the decline of intellectual and physical ability." According to the brochure—which seems at least to have Aslan's tacit endorsement, since her name and face are displayed prominently—GH-3 can cure every age-related illness from wrinkles, ulcers, and a condition dubbed "neurovegetative discordance" to arthritis, heart attacks, and Parkinson's disease.

Although she's somewhat more scientific than the Bucharest travel agents, Ana Aslan is no less enthusiastic in her claims for what GH-3 can do. When she came to the United States in 1973 to help the Food and Drug Administration set up its first clinical trials testing the value of

GH-3 in geriatric depression—the only claim for which the scientific community was willing to give the drug an edge—Aslan was a sprightly seventy-six years old. She was described as "a walking advertisement for her treatment." Aslan told a reporter for *Medical World News* that, while GH-3's antidepressant activity may be what finally gets the drug marketed in the United States, its other benefits would no doubt soon become evident. "I am confident that physicians watching patients treated [for depression] with our drug will be impressed by their overall physical as well as mental improvement," she said. In 145 gerontology clinics in Romania, Aslan added, hundreds of middle-aged persons were receiving GH-3 to ward off old age, and 70 percent of them showed "improvement in psychic condition, work capacity, appetite and weight, morbidity rate, and resistance to stress."

The FDA's depression trials indicated that GH-3 might indeed have a place in today's medical marketplace. The drug seemed better able to reverse the symptoms of depression in the aged in several carefully designed studies than did placebos given to control groups of patients. And perhaps more convincing were the basic animal studies conducted concurrently with clinical trials that showed the antidepressant effects of GH-3 at the cellular level.

As we saw in chapter 2, one of the few neurotransmitters known to increase in the brain with age is MAO—monoamine oxidase, an acknowledged "disaster" of a neurotransmitter whose presence makes an individual susceptible to clinical depression. Recent attempts at treatment of depression have included the use of a class of drugs known as MAO inhibitors—pargyline, phenelzine, and tranylcypromine, for example. These drugs have serious side effects, though, especially if the patient has recently taken drugs in another category of antidepressants, the tricyclics, or if he eats foods containing tyramine (such as cheese or wine) or takes medications containing sympathomimetic amines (such as many popular cold preparations).

Gerovital H-3 appears to be an effective MAO inhibitor that has none of the serious side effects of the drugs now in use in this country. At the University of Southern California, gerontologist Josef P. Hrachovec found that GH-3, when administered to rats, reduced the level of MAO in the brain by 43 percent after just twenty minutes. Within thirty minutes, the MAO level was reduced by 51 percent, and, when the concentration of GH-3 delivered to the rats was increased, reductions as high as 87 percent were achieved. The great benefit of GH-3 over the other MAO inhibitors is that its action is more selective, so that GH-3 does not interfere, as the others do, with the metabolic work of the liver. This makes GH-3 free of a side effect of the MAO inhibitors that renders those drugs especially hazardous to the aged—their tendency to bring on toxic hypertensive crisis, an extremely high blood pressure due to inadequate elimination of toxic compounds called amines.

From Self-Help to Small Help: The Anti-Senility Drugs

If self-administered nutrients, vitamins, and potions seem to offer little assistance in warding off the mental changes of old age, prescription drugs dispensed by doctors sometimes seem to offer even less. Physicians are unaccustomed to dealing with diseases for which there is no easy remedy; in the 1980s the usual method of treating any condition, from a common cold to menopause, is to prescribe a pill, whether it is needed or not. But Alzheimer's disease defies this remedy.

Scores of clinical trials have been undertaken in the last

decade to see which of several promising drugs might help clear the mental haze that often accompanies Alzheimer's disease. Some of these drugs occasionally improve intellectual functioning in patients with senile dementia; others sometimes help in terms of mood, orientation, attitude, ability to feed and dress oneself, or other behavioral factors. When all the studies are looked at as a whole, however, there are enough inconsistencies and contradictory findings almost to cancel out any positive conclusions. To date, the most beneficial drug for Alzheimer's disease seems to be the vasodilator Hydergine, and the most promising drug of the future the nootropic Piracetam. But these drugs are useful, not because they "cure" senile dementia, but only because they clear up certain symptoms — which is more than can be said for most other "anti-senility" drugs.

Once again, the drugs we will review in this section — primarily Hydergine, L-dopa, chelating agents, centrophenoxine, and Piracetam — have *not* been shown unequivocally to benefit Alzheimer's disease patients or even to minimize the cognitive changes of old age. They are not described here so that patients can begin haranguing their doctors for a prescription; indeed, many of them are only available on an experimental basis to qualified scientist-investigators. The drugs we will look at are offered as an indication of the research flurry now underway in the race to find a treatment for Alzheimer's disease — and the flurry, if nothing else, should be of some comfort for the disease's victims and their families.

ANTI-SENILITY DRUGS, I: THE VASODILATORS

It's been years since the leaders of the medical community have equated "senility" with "hardening of the arteries of the brain." The message has begun to trickle down even to the family physician that senile dementia usually is not a vascular problem, but is, by and large, a neurological disease. Nonetheless, some scientists have been trying to correct the symptoms of senile dementia with drugs that work directly on expanding the blood vessels in the brain, thereby increasing blood circulation to the neurons. This group of drugs is called vasodilators. Oddly enough, even though the blood vessels in Alzheimer's disease and other forms of senile dementia usually are not clogged, vasodilators seem to have at least some beneficial effect on impaired memory, orientation, and thought processes.

The most popular of the vasodilators is Hydergine. In California, Hydergine is ranked number two, after the tranquilizer Mellaril, in total drug expenditures among the institutionalized aged. But just because a drug is popular doesn't necessarily mean it works. Hydergine has been tested in several clinical trials to compare its effects with those of another vasodilator, papaverine, and those of a placebo pill. In most studies, Hydergine came out the winner—but only by a nose. John R. Hughes of the University of Mississippi Medical Center, who reviewed the findings of twelve of those clinical trials conducted between 1969 and 1975, concluded that "because of the small magnitude of the improvement and the absence of indications of long-term benefit, Hydergine would seem to be of minor value in dementia therapy."

Still, for the time being, Hydergine seems to be almost all there is. Physicians and patients feel better when some sort of drug is prescribed at the end of a doctor's appointment, so the prescription written these days when a patient has Alzheimer's disease is often for Hydergine. At least Hydergine makes many patients more alert, more sociable, less anxious—behavioral measures that are important in making a patient with senile dementia more independent and easier to care for. Unfortunately, no one is claiming that Hydergine has any benefit in the areas that most concern Alzheimer's disease victims: memory and cognition.

One study conducted at several nursing homes in Germany is perhaps more optimistic than the others regarding the therapeutic value of Hydergine. J. Kugler and his associates gave Hydergine to a group of nursing home residents, and a placebo to a similar group who acted as controls. Neither patients nor physicians knew which group was receiving which drug; this experimental design is known as a double-blind controlled clinical trial. After six months of daily doses of 4.5 milligrams of Hydergine, the treated group showed no improvement over the control group. But after fifteen months of therapy, the treated group showed an average of 5 to 7 percent increase in test scores for general intelligence, while the control subjects declined in these scores. The findings are, as the physicians say, suggestive.

Physicians prescribe Hydergine based in part on findings such as Kugler's, and in part on the knowledge that the drug has been prescribed for long-term therapy for many years with no apparent side effects. If it leads to some improvement, the reasoning is, it is worth a try, so long as it doesn't seem to hurt the patient. But one continuing problem with the drug is that it is offered most commonly in a tablet that cannot be swallowed, but must be taken sublingually—that is, by dissolving it under the tongue. This method can prove difficult for patients already suffering from confusion and forgetfulness, and studies are underway to convert Hydergine to a form that is easier to take at home.

Hydergine is not the only vasodilator on the market

that has been used to treat senile dementia. A series of other drugs has been tried, too, such as Cyclospasmol, Vasodilan, papaverine, and, in Europe, Surheme, Trental, Praxilene, and Sermon. Some have been shown beneficial to patients with Alzheimer's disease. But this fact, says Boston pharmacologist Roland Branconnier, presents "a conceptual problem. If [the drugs] really work by dilating brain arteries or arterioles, should this effect be helpful?" For one thing, cerebral arteriosclerosis does not seem to be a factor in the vast majority of senile dementia cases. For another thing, it is unlikely that vasodilators are really having much effect on already hardened arteries, which have lost most of their elasticity; therefore, only the normal arteries are expanded by the drug's action, which we might expect to aggravate, not ease, the problem for the diseased part of the brain by making it easier for blood to flow only to the healthier regions. Branconnier and his colleague, Jonathan Cole of McLean Hospital in Belmont, Massachusetts, offer a theory to explain this apparent paradox: "Vasodilators may dilate capillaries," the tiny blood vessels not affected by arteriosclerosis, they suggest, "or increase the deformability of red blood cells [that is, their ability to squeeze through narrower vessels], and thus improve the tissue blood supply." In addition, some vasodilators may have other effects that are important in the treatment of Alzheimer's disease. Hydergine, for example, is known to improve the brain's ability to metabolize glucose and to utilize oxygen, two steps essential for the viability of mental functioning.

ANTI-SENILITY DRUGS, II: L-DOPA

Parkinson's disease is a neurological disorder affecting less than 1 percent of the population. Like Alzheimer's disease, it tends to be a disease of old age, though it can strike persons in their middle years. It is characterized most dramatically by involuntary shaking and eventual stiffening of the limbs and head, but its other symptoms include mental debilities that look very much like senility.

Patients with senile dementia, conversely, often exhibit mild symptoms that doctors call Parkinson-like: trembling, shaking, shuffling, nodding, mumbling. This link between Parkinson's and Alzheimer's disease has been strengthened on autopsy studies of the brains of patients who died with either of the two disorders: in each group, an unusual number of neuritic plaques have been found.

Parkinson's disease is one of the success stories of medicine in the 1970s. Early in the decade, neurologist George Cotzias discovered that Parkinson's patients seemed to be missing an essential enzyme—levodopa—used in the manufacture of the neurotransmitter dopamine. Dopamine is part of a group of transmitters called catecholamines, of which acetylcholine is also a part. When the missing levodopa was replaced in Parkinson's patients with an identical drug, the physical symptoms of Parkinsonism, as well as some of the mental changes, began to disappear. Today, L-dopa allows many patients with Parkinson's disease to live relatively normal, symptom-free lives.

Martin Albert, a neurologist at Boston University, studied the mental changes that accompany Parkinson's disease and plotted them on a chart, recording scores on tests of language skills, perception, memory, rate of information processing, and other measures. He then administered the same tests to two other groups of people: those with Huntington's disease, another neurological disorder that also leads to mental decay; and normal elderly persons. The shape of the Parkinson's disease curve was almost identical to the normal aged group's. Later, Albert checked the pattern of dementia in Alzheimer's disease, too, and found that it did not correlate with normal aging nearly as well as Parkinson's disease did. He called Parkinson's disease a "subcortical dementia"—a neurological disease process affecting not the cortex, as Alzheimer's disease does, but the cerebrum and cerebellum—and theorized that aging itself may be a "slowly progressive subcortical dementia."

If Parkinson's disease and normal aging produce the same kind of mental changes—characterized by Albert as inertia, apathy, memory dysfunction, inability to use new knowledge, and slowness in the rate of information processing—can the dramatic new cure for Parkinson's disease be used to cure the mental changes of age? Several scientists thinking along these lines have tried L-dopa in elderly patients with mild to moderate memory impairment, as well as in those with diagnosed Alzheimer's disease. The results, like so many in this field, have been equivocal. At New York University, for example, Steven Ferris and his colleagues tried L-dopa in sixteen mildly to moderately impaired aged individuals. After four weeks, the scientists noted some changes in mood and cognitive test performance, "but no consistent pattern of improvement." Another group of patients treated by David Drachman at Northwestern University fared better, however: These slightly impaired patients, who exhibited mild physical symptoms of Parkinsonism along with their dementia, improved both physically and mentally after treatment with L-dopa. But a group of Scandinavian scientists conducting a more careful, placebo-control study noted no advantage for L-dopa over a placebo in a group of patients with pre-senile dementia.

Allan S. Presly and his colleagues at the Royal Dundee Liff Hospital in Scotland were even more equivocal in their findings about L-dopa. The psychologists tested the drug on fourteen very old women (with an average age of almost seventy-nine) suffering from senile dementia, and after four weeks of therapy noted a significant improvement in intellectual functioning, an improvement that was "quite striking in some patients" and very clear in at least ten of the fourteen. Although L-dopa did not improve any of the behavioral indices measured other than communication and continence—meaning that the level of mobility, orientation, cooperation, restlessness, mood, and independence basically remained the same or worsened—the scientists noted that "any agent that may produce benefit to this virtually untreatable condition is of interest and worthy of further investigation."

Presly made his report in the March 1978 issue of the *British Medical Journal.* In June he and his colleagues published the results of a follow-up study, in which L-dopa therapy had been continued for an additional six months (after a one-month break following the original study). Intellectual performance scores had declined during the drug-free layover, they noted, but improved once again when L-dopa therapy was begun and, by the end of the six months, "were comparable to the scores during the active preparation phase of the original trial." But the psychologists made a disturbing finding: Of the five patients in this extended phase of the study, only three showed intellectual improvement, while one progressively deteriorated and the fifth exhibited "a very spectacular decline in functioning between the last two [monthly] ratings." The conclusion of Presly's group as of June 1978 was: "We are doubtful whether levodopa should be recommended for the routine treatment of this condition at present." As with so many other treatments, physicians cannot even agree with each other—or, sometimes, with their own prior conclusions—and patients are left totally in the dark as to what approach is best.

ANTI-SENILITY DRUGS, III: CHELATION THERAPY

One issue physicians—at least those in the medical mainstream—agree on is that chelation therapy is quackery.
Chelation, from the Greek word for "claw," is the process
by which one metallic ion clamps onto another and drags
the metal out of the body. Chelating agents originally were
developed as an antidote to lead and other metal intoxication, but in the past decade some have claimed it can cure
atherosclerosis by dragging cholesterol deposits out of the
body, too. The American Medical Association (AMA) has
compiled documents and articles for distribution to practi-
tioners assuring them that chelating agents can do nothing
to cure atherosclerosis. "There are several sites in the
United States and Canada where this therapeutic fad cur-
rently is in vogue and where the zealot peddles these wares
to the naive afflicted," wrote Alfred Soffer of the Chicago
Medical School in the *Journal of the AMA*. "Symposia and
mini-conventions have been organized to extol its virtues.
Publicity attendant to these events has resulted in an increasing number of inquiries to those of us who have studied basic concepts of metal binding. We have been startled
and chagrined in recent times to learn that a number of
physicians ascribe to this drug an efficacy that has not been
established by fundamental clinical investigation."

Chelating agents counteract the harm done by toxic
levels of lead or other heavy metals, such as mercury, by
binding with the metal and thus removing large quantities
of it from the bloodstream. Many chelating agents, such as
disodium edetate (known by the brand name Endrate), bind
with calcium as well as metals, making them dangerous to
use in cases of metal poisoning because they could damage
bone tissue before cleaning out the metal.

In the early 1970s, though, some scientists began to

wonder whether Endrate's calcium-binding capacity could be used to advantage. They hypothesized that the drug could wash away the fat deposits that accumulate in blood vessels with atherosclerosis. At a cost of from $20 to $100 a treatment, some medical clinics began offering chelation therapy as a "life-saving and sometimes miraculous" cure for hardening of the arteries. A typical treatment course runs up to thirty treatments, which could cost an individual as much as $3,000 for a procedure that has not yet been proved. Because of the money involved and the expectations that might be dashed, the AMA set out to discredit the value of chelation therapy.

But in 1979 pharmacologists Roland Branconnier and Jonathan Cole of Massachusetts suggested that chelation therapy in the treatment of certain ailments of old age might not be quackery after all. Proposing what they admitted was a "radical treatment approach," Branconnier and Cole said some chelating agents might be useful in the treatment of Alzheimer's disease. They cited abundant evidence that chronic accumulation of aluminum in the brain could lead to the neurofibrillary tangles typical of Alzheimer's disease (as the work of Donald Crapper McLachlan and others has shown), and said chelators might be useful in binding aluminum and removing it from the neurons. They urged animal studies to see whether this approach makes clinical sense. If the experiments bear out Branconnier and Cole's hypothesis, perhaps human studies could be begun within the next few years.

ANTI-SENILITY DRUGS, IV: CENTROPHENOXINE

Another drug that seems almost too good to be true—and is therefore met with some skepticism by the medical establishment—is centrophenoxine. This compound, which is known to stimulate glucose metabolism, oxygen consumption, and carbon dioxide production in the brain (all related to the brain's level of activation), has been found in rats to produce a remarkable change: Long-term therapy with centrophenoxine seems to wash away lipofuscin, the age pigment found in the brain, heart, and other tissues of animals and humans as they age.

Kalidas Nandy of Boston University is a leader in experimentation with centrophenoxine. He and his colleagues have been finding not only that the amount of lipofuscin diminishes and sometimes disappears in old animals given centrophenoxine, but that these treated animals seem to live longer, too. And in experiments with mice, some scientists have found that the animals treated with centrophenoxine have an increased learning capacity compared with the untreated animals.

One biologist, I. Zs.-Nagy of the Medical University of Debrecen, has gone so far as to speculate that centrophenoxine may be an effective "anti-aging drug." On the basis of the "membrane hypothesis of cellular aging" that he developed in 1978, Zs.-Nagy theorized that centrophenoxine may act not only on age pigments but on the underlying mechanism of aging itself.

According to the membrane hypothesis, an essential change that occurs during aging is the increasing rigidity of the membrane encasing the cell. As the cell membrane becomes more rigid, it becomes more impervious to the ions that must pass through into the cell in order for life processes to continue. Potassium ions ordinarily pass from the intercellular space into the cell body; the concentration within the cell of potassium ions, in turn, stimulates the RNA to transcribe its genetic information and to manufacture protein—an essential process of life. If potassium ions cannot pass through the cell membrane of older cells,

Zs.-Nagy theorizes, the cell maintains a higher concentration of potassium ions within the cell body to "compensate for the decrease of potassium permeability of the cell membrane, so that the cell remains excitable even in old age." But at the same time that the high potassium concentration is keeping the cell excitable, it is also debilitating the functioning of RNA, which is highly sensitive to ionic strength and cannot transcribe information properly when the concentration of potassium ions gets too high. The result: a serious decrease in the aged cell's ability to synthesize protein.

Centrophenoxine, Zs.-Nagy theorizes, may have a "membrane affinity," meaning it attaches itself to the cell membrane and alters its permeability. If the membrane returns to its youthful state of allowing the free flow of potassium ions, the ionic balance within the cell can return to a normal level, and the production of protein can continue.

"Under such circumstances, the nerve cells are able to eliminate the accumulated aging pigments," Zs.-Nagy says. "This may be due either to an increased lysosomal enzyme synthesis [an enzyme needed to metabolize lipofuscin], or a decreased rate of lipofuscin production, or even to both." Whatever the mechanism, the consensus is building that centrophenoxine appears to wash out some of the cellular damage of old age, especially in the brain. The next step is clinical trials, conducted on aged individuals simply complaining of memory loss and confusion, or diagnosed as having Alzheimer's disease; such trials should help scientists discover whether the established effects of centrophenoxine at the cellular level make any difference in terms of an individual's mental functioning. At least one leading scientist thinks that it won't. Centrophenoxine probably does clean out lipofuscin deposits, notes Edward Schneider, scientific director of the NIA. But lipofuscin might not do any damage in the first place. "Human cells, such as the neurons of the inferior olivary nucleus, accumulate large amounts of . . . lipofuscin," Schneider says, "yet neuronal loss in this [region of the brain] is not detected even into the ninth decade. Therefore, although accumulation of these large pigments with aging is impressive, it may have little functional impact."

ANTI-SENILITY DRUGS, V: NOOTROPICS

In 1972 the Belgian pharmacologist C. Giurgea discovered a new class of drugs. He called the compounds "nootropics," from the Greek word *noos*, for "mind," and *tropein*, for "toward." As Giurgea defined it, nootropics seemed made to order for correcting the cognitive problems of aging: they act specifically on the brain's integrative and associative mechanisms and have few peripheral effects on other systems of the body.

The term "nootropic" has been loosely applied since then to any drug thought to heighten mental sharpness in old age. But only a few drugs accurately fit Giurgea's original definition. The most popular and promising one is called Piracetam. A number of studies have been conducted recently, but Piracetam still is available in the United States only on an experimental basis. The manufacturer, Parke-Davis, also has several other nootropics under study, known by code names such as CI (for "clinical investigation") 844, CI 879, CI 911, and CI 933.

Pharmacologists call Piracetam an "odd drug." Chemically, its structure is unusual; it consists of a neurotransmitter, GABA (gamma-amino-butyric acid), that has been curled into a ring from its usual chain configuration. Piracetam has been shown to improve learning ability in animals, to delay amnesia usually brought about by oxygen deprivation, and, perhaps most important, to change the electroencephalogram (EEG) pattern in a way that confirms scientists' belief that, in man, the drug enhances associative processing in the cortex and facilitates the transfer of information from one brain hemisphere to the other.

Unlike other drugs that affect the central nervous system, Piracetam has no pain-killing, sedating, or tranquilizing effect. This can prove to be especially beneficial to the aged, who are more sensitive than others to the side effects that usually accompany psychoactive drugs.

Early clinical studies of the drug are encouraging. When 400 milligrams of Piracetam were given daily to a group of healthy college students for two weeks, the students showed a significantly improved ability to memorize a specific series of words. In an older group of healthy adults complaining of memory loss, another researcher found that 1.6 grams of Piracetam a day improved both cognitive performance and psychiatric impressions of the subjects as recorded by a psychiatrist and a psychologist. The nineteen subjects in this study ranged in age from forty-seven to seventy-three. Finally, 2.4 grams of Piracetam given daily to a group of impaired elderly persons classified as having mild, moderate, or severe dementia led to a significant improvement in the mildly and moderately demented groups in such variables as fatigue, understanding, attention, concentration, irritability, agitation, and circumstantiality. The severely demented patients, however, failed to respond to the Piracetam.

Knowledge of Piracetam's physiological action and evidence of its clinical success have led traditionally skeptical physicians to some guarded optimism about the nootropics as a useful anti-senility compound. "We may conclude at this time that Piracetam is an interesting and seemingly unique substance," say Steven Ferris and his colleagues at New York University, "which may be the forerunner of a new pharmacologic class of compounds. There is preliminary evidence that it may be useful in improving functioning in patients with mild to moderate senile dementia." That's as hopeful an endorsement as any other drug has yet received in the generally bleak therapeutic landscape of Alzheimer's disease.

The Physical Therapies: Cure by Manipulation

Investigations into possible means of treating Alzheimer's disease and mental changes of age have taken a third tack as well: attempts to restore cognition through manipulation. If nutrients and prescription drugs don't work, perhaps a more physical, structurally oriented approach will.

The history of such attempts has been disappointing. Great excitement was created more than a decade ago when two physical therapies for senile dementia—hyperbaric oxygenation and cerebro-ventricular shunts—seemed to bring about miraculous improvement in experimental subjects. But the excitement waned when, in the case of hyperbaric oxygenation, the dramatic results could not be replicated, and when, in the case of brain shunts, the procedure was applied indiscriminately to patients who should not have received it.

Today most such manipulations have been discredited, or are applied only to a very carefully defined group of patients, and therefore are not likely to become the Alzheimer's cure of tomorrow. But around the corner may be some lesser known, homier kinds of physical approaches to the problem—such as those utilized by the Friendship Center of New York City or the SAGE program (Senior Actualization and Growth Exploration) of Berkeley, California—that could prove at least to alleviate the discomforts and disabilities of senile dementia, and make the final years for many people, impaired or relatively unimpaired, fuller and more independent.

THE PHYSICAL THERAPIES, I: HIGH-PRESSURE OXYGEN

Eleanor Jacobs, a psychiatrist at the Buffalo (New York) Veterans Administration Hospital, caused quite a stir in the medical world in 1969. She reported that she could significantly improve the mental functioning of old, forgetful men by administering pure oxygen to them at twice the normal pressure of the atmosphere. The oxygen was breathed in a huge chamber, called a hyperbaric (high-pressure) chamber, through a full-face mask. After two ninety-minute sessions daily for fifteen days, Jacobs made a report in the widely read *New England Journal of Medicine*. The thirteen men she studied, she said, all of whom suffered severe mental deterioration, were "markedly and reliably" improved in terms of performance on memory function tests. On the Wechsler Memory Scale, for example, the experimental subjects jumped from a mean score of 76 before treatment to 103 afterward—a statistically significant improvement. In contrast, a group of five control subjects, who breathed ordinary air in the high-pressure chamber instead of breathing pure oxygen, barely changed their scores, compiling a pre-treatment average of 80 and an average of 78 after treatment. But when the control subjects were placed on the experimental group's regimen—receiving 100 percent oxygen at high pressures twice daily, for ninety minutes a session, for fifteen days—their memory scores jumped, too, to an average of 100.

"It is not likely that the treatment modifies basic degenerative processes," wrote Jacobs and her colleagues in describing these findings, "but we know of no other form of therapy that offers statistically significant improvement of function. The value of such symptomatic benefit will depend largely on its duration (after the treatment series ends) and whether a retreatment schedule will maintain the effect. Both aspects remain to be investigated."

Several of Jacobs's peers accepted her invitation to investigate further the dramatic results she had achieved. Although her experiment, which used a group of control subjects, was considered a well-designed test, it could not be reproduced by the investigators who tried to do so using the same experimental design. In four uncontrolled studies, though, certain improvements were noted after hyperoxygenation. One scientist who joined the attempt to reproduce Jacobs's findings, Alvin Goldfarb of Mount Sinai Medical School in New York, ran into an unexpected problem in his own study. Although his subjects, many of them Jewish immigrants, had severe memory problems, their memory of one period of their lives was sharp and painful enough still to render them incapable of participating in the experiment: The hyperbaric oxygen chamber reminded them of the Nazi gas chambers, and they could not bring themselves to step inside.

Even though the scientific confirmation of Jacobs's wonder therapy was at best equivocal, more and more hospitals began installing, and using, hyperbaric oxygenation chambers of their own. As Jacobs and her colleagues had implied in their 1969 article, something, or even the hope of something, is better than nothing—and nothing was all that institutions at the time were offering their senile patients. The National Institute of Mental Health (NIMH), however, was distressed by the possible expenditure of thousands of wasted dollars (fifteen sessions in the chamber, in the early 1970s, cost approximately $900, and were usually repeated six months later), and it embarked on a study of its own. In collaboration with Samuel Gershon and his colleagues at New York University, NIMH psychopharmacologist Allen Raskin and psychotherapist Thomas Crook investigated the value of hyperbaric oxygen in the treatment of senile symptoms.

The NIMH study used 82 carefully selected subjects who were intact enough to live in the community, yet who revealed memory losses more severe than one would expect for their age. The subjects, whose average age was seventy-two, were divided into four groups of approximately equal size, randomly assigned to receive either high-pressure oxygen, high-pressure air, normal-pressure oxygen, or normal-pressure air during the ninety-minute sessions scheduled twice daily for fifteen days. The aim of the study design was to see whether any changes in mental performance before and after treatment could be detected, and then to see whether the degree of pressure (high versus normal) or the substance delivered (oxygen versus normal air) was the factor that made the difference.

As it turned out, nothing made a difference at all. "Simply put, the results of this study failed to sustain the view that oxygen treatment, under either hyperbaric, or normobaric conditions, has beneficial effects on cognitive impairment in the elderly." And, contrary to Goldfarb's findings of intense anxiety generated by the association of the hyperbaric chamber with Nazi gas chambers, the NIMH group found that the mystique of the chamber, which inside resembles "a spaceship or a submarine," created what they called a "halo effect." Patients who received either air or oxygen in the high-pressure chamber seemed to *feel* better than those who had received their treatment in a hospital room at normal pressures. They reported feeling less anxious, less depressed, and less fatigued after fifteen days of treatment than they had been before. The aura of stepping into a high-technology cure vessel seemed to have done a better job of helping them than did the treatment itself.

THE PHYSICAL THERAPIES, II: BRAIN SHUNTING

It seemed almost a miracle cure. Several patients, each of them complaining of the same general symptoms — forgetfulness, unsteady gait and frequent falling, inability to concentrate, occasional incontinence — came to the Massachusetts General Hospital and perplexed the entire staff. The patients didn't seem to have any physical problems that could explain the symptoms. There was no indication of infection, heart disease, metabolic disease, drug toxicity, or any of the other causes of treatable "pseudosenility" discussed in chapter 4. Their brain X rays appeared normal, and the tests used to determine the level of pressure in the cerebrospinal fluid — which cushions the brain and spine in an intricate shock absorber system — seemed normal, too. The doctors were just about to make the final diagnosis: senile dementia.

But the results of one brain test proved troubling enough to make the doctors think one more time before calling the disease incurable. When the patients were given a pneumoencephalogram — in which air is forced into the brain to allow an X ray to reveal the structure of the brain — an oddity turned up. In each of these patients, the ventricles, the four fluid-filled spaces in the brain that are an essential part of the shock absorber system, had swelled enormously. If the ventricles are so large, the physicians reasoned, there must be an excess buildup of fluid within them. And they theorized that a previously unknown condition, hydrocephalus in the aged, had been discovered.

Hydrocephalus (from the Greek words for "water" and "brain") had been known to occur in infants due to a congenital malformation in the skull. Because infants' skulls are relatively soft during the first year of life, their heads are able to enlarge to accommodate the excess fluid that collects in the ventricles. And because of this head enlargement, physicians can easily spot a hydrocephalic child, and save it from the lifetime of severe mental and physical deterioration that would occur if the fluid accumulation continued unchecked.

What doctors do is this: They drill a tiny hole in the child's skull, insert a microscopic tube into a ventricle, and run the tube under the scalp and neck skin into the jugular vein of the neck. From there, the tube continues into a chamber of the heart, where it can drain as part of the fluid circulation of the heart itself. The operation is considered relatively simple, and its results are remarkable.

On the assumption that the elderly patients at Massachusetts General Hospital had a similar condition, their physicians, led by Raymond Adams, performed a similar operation—a ventriculo-atrial shunt. Within weeks, the patients had improved dramatically. One, a sixty-two-year-old pediatrician, was back at work treating his patients and feeling fit as ever; another, a sixty-three-year-old woman, was soon performing at a "superior" and "very superior" level on tests of intellectual skill and memory functioning.

Adams's team reported its success in 1965, and coined a new word for the condition: "normal pressure hydrocephalus." Because the aged patient's brain fluid pressure does not increase, the disease is a tricky one to detect, and Adams emphasized that three symptoms must be present for an operation even to be considered: forgetfulness, unsteady gait, and urinary incontinence. Then, a test to determine the size of the ventricles must be performed (in 1965 the typical test used was the painful, and sometimes dangerous, pneumonecephalogram; today newer techniques such as cisternography and CT scans are available). If all three symptoms are present and if the ventricles are enlarged, Adams estimates that 50 percent of ventriculo-atrial shunts performed will be successful in reversing the condition.

Adams's estimate is a cautious one, but it hasn't fazed the zealous. Eager for the chance of a dramatic, instantaneous cure for an apparently hopeless state, doctors and patients alike have overused the brain shunt procedure in recent years. "I don't think any of these things are ever maliciously contrived," says neurologist Howard Hurtig of the Graduate Hospital of the University of Pennsylvania. "I don't think doctors go out and put shunts in people's brains because they have a demonic view of brain function. They really think they're going to help people—but they get a little bit carried away, and they let their subjective sense of things interfere with their scientific detachment. They'll shunt somebody and say, 'My God, he's so much better,' and the family will say, 'Yes, he really is better,' and they all convince themselves."

Scientists who have tried to measure post-shunting improvement in some objective way have generally been unable to prove that the operation clearly leads to improved functioning. Hurtig likens the once-popular diagnosis of normal pressure hydrocephalus to the Cheshire Cat in *Alice in Wonderland*: "The more we understand, the less it appears to be a real thing." With this caveat, and with the 50-50 odds that a cautious physician such as Adams offers for carefully screened surgical candidates, scientists hesitate to call the brain shunt anything but an outside chance for returned functioning for a very few apparent victims of senile dementia.

THE PHYSICAL THERAPIES, III: ENVIRONMENTAL BOOSTS

Sometimes the simplest changes made the biggest differences. Shunning the high-technology senility "fixes" of hyperbaric chambers and operating rooms, a handful of therapists have tried some old-fashioned ways of helping old people maintain their mental functioning for as long as possible. The methods are disarmingly simple, borrowed from methods used instinctively in the family network when one family member is more important than the rest. The therapists are trying to do what a loving son or daughter would do for an ailing parent: give him the time, support, and assistance he needs to do things for himself.

At the Friendship Center in New York City, for example, a "drop-in" social lounge is open three afternoons a week for the old people in the surrounding Lower East Side community. During those afternoons, nothing happens. The old people are free to sit alone or in small groups, to drink coffee or watch television or stare at the empty wall. If they want to consult with staff members for help in understanding a phone bill or obtaining a welfare check, they may. But if they suggest organizing a game of bingo or a sing-along, they are told to go somewhere else. Persons who need such activities don't belong at the Friendship Center; the Friendship Center is for the "frail elderly" for whom such activities would be a threat.

Ironically, the deliberately low-key environment of the place seems to be what many of these people need in order to come out of themselves. There are regulars at the Friendship Center, just as there are at centers where something is always happening, but they come here not for sociability but for solace. "There is no pressure to participate," gerontologist Janet Sainer told the Gerontological Society at its 1977 meeting. "People are able to sit and rest quietly, with others or alone, comfortable in the knowledge that the staff welcomes and accepts them as they are, is aware of their presence, and is available for help when needed." The predictability of an afternoon in the lounge is a great comfort to these people, she said, as is their knowledge that they may sit, nap, stare, without any obligation to return a smile or answer a question. "We found that any changes, even the rearrangement of furniture, generates a great deal of anxiety," she said. But the proximity of the staff members, and the lack of pressure to form a relationship with them, enables the more withdrawn among the clientele gradually to talk about their problems and to accept help when it is offered.

Just slightly more engaged than the approach used at the Friendship Center is a technique called reality orientation. This was introduced by James Folsom, medical director of the Veterans Administration Hospital in Tuscaloosa, Alabama, in the mid-1960s, and once again is a formalization of what many family members probably do instinctively. As used now at nursing homes and other long-term care facilities around the country, reality orientation is a way of bringing confused, disoriented old men and women back to the real world. Visual and verbal clues as to time and place are repeated over and over: calendars, clocks, and bulletin boards are prominently displayed so that residents know precisely what day it is, what time it is, and what the next meal is. If someone wakes in the middle of the night calling for his mother, he is told his name, that his mother's been dead for thirty years, and that it's three hours till breakfast. If someone staring out the window murmurs, "I see a pink cow," she is told to look again until she realizes the pink she sees is a car. Some institutions go so far as to hold regular reality orientation classes, where the basic facts of everyday life are repeated again and again. Staff members are instructed to call each resident by name—a simple courtesy often overlooked in nursing homes, which can contribute to a resident's confusion as to who he or she is. Since Folsom first coined the term, reality orientation has been used in one form or another in almost every nursing home in America. Because all staff members, from medical director to orderly, are involved in the technique—which requires round-the-clock reinforcement—one of its most tangible benefits is that it infuses the staff with positive feelings toward the nursing home residents, feelings that translate into smiles, assistance, gestures, and words that had been missing before. It is impossible to separate the benefit of human kindness from the advantage of being told, over and over, your name and the day of the week.

A third type of environmental therapy, which takes as its starting point this universal need for human kindness, is the SAGE program. SAGE, an acronym for "senior actualization and growth experience," borrows techniques from Eastern religion, biofeedback, the California-inspired human potential movement, and old-fashioned physical therapy to restore old people to optimal functioning, and to help them approach the final stage of life as a time of continued growth and self-exploration.

"People could grow as much at seventy-five as at twenty-five," says SAGE founder Gay Luce, a Berkeley psychologist, "if given the same conditions that inspire growth in the young—nurturance, support, challenge, freedom, and continued activity." In what has been described as a "mini-Esalen for the aging." SAGE encourages participants to learn techniques of relaxation, to use their bodies in new ways (for example, through the rigorous, stylized move-

209

ments of Tai Chi), and to explore their feelings about life and death. The SAGE program has been taken successfully to nursing homes as well, where, says SAGE co-founder Eugenia Gerrard, "there are few opportunities for residents to explore their potential for growth and change, to experience the depth of their feelings, or to talk about their concerns. By their structure and purpose, institutions serving the aged encourage their clients to 'rest' or 'convalesce,' engendering feelings of uselessness." Through group meetings that include anything from personal recollections to mild physical exercise to arguments over the day's current events, SAGE volunteers manage to bring nursing home residents out of their shells. Says Gerrard: "People look forward to meeting with us and talking about themselves, people who otherwise sleep most of the day."

In chapter 9, we shall look at other ways in which the environment, both inside and outside the institution, can be modified to encourage the aged to operate to their fullest capacity. We shall explore the "Environmental Docility Hypothesis," which says that the less competent the individuals, the more they are affected—either positively or negatively—by changes in the environment. But first we shall look, in the following chapter, at the individual who perhaps has more to say about the quality of an old person's surroundings than any other single individual, except perhaps a spouse or a son or daughter: the old person's physician. And we shall see why doctors have a lot to learn before it can be said that they understand the particular needs and strengths of their patients over the age of sixty-five.

•*8*•

Medical Ageism

Robert Butler, when he was director of the National Institute on Aging (NIA), often told the story of his old friend Morris Rocklin. When Rocklin was 101 years old, he went to see his doctor, complaining of pain in his left leg. "Morris, for Pete's sake, what do you expect at 101?" his doctor said. Shot back Morris: "Look, my right leg is also 101, but it doesn't hurt a bit. Now explain that!"

Butler, now chairman of the Department of Geriatrics and Adult Development at the Mount Sinai Medical Center at New York, told the story to illustrate the unconscious ageism that even the most well-intentioned doctors can reveal in their dealings with the old. Morris Rocklin was too feisty to settle for a shrug of the shoulders and a reassurance of "You're just no spring chicken anymore." But countless old people, themselves believing that aches and pains and incapacities are part of old age, leave their physicians' offices daily with just such non-diagnoses. The result may be thousands of missed cases of disorders that are not part of normal aging, but are illnesses that can be treated and cured. No one knows how many of today's elderly are suffering needlessly simply because they, or their families, or their doctors, shrugged and said, "Well, what do you expect?"

Everyone over the age of sixty-five, the healthy as well as the infirm, is hurt when the myth of senility quietly pervades the doctor's office. With 85 percent of elderly Americans suffering from at least one chronic disorder, and more commonly two or three, even the relatively fit and independent old person must make frequent trips to the doctor and receive frequent doses of the "therapeutic nihilism" that characterizes many doctors' treatment of the old. These physicians approach their aged patients with the belief that disability is inevitable, pain is expected, and senility is acceptable. And this belief has profound implications for the quality of care they can deliver.

In some instances, the belief can lead physicians to take actions that are actually harmful to the elderly. Physician Richard Shannon remembers one such scene in a hospital intensive-care unit (ICU) which he witnessed in 1979 as a medical student at the University of Connecticut. Mrs. Goode (not her real name), an alert, well-read, pleasant eighty-two-year-old woman, was recovering uneventfully from the successful removal of a lung tumor. But eighteen hours after surgery, still in intensive care, Mrs. Goode began to shout incoherently, thrashing about and tearing at her tubes. Had she been forty-two years old, the ICU staff—who did not know the patient—would have looked quickly for a physical explanation for her sudden bout of "craziness." But she was eighty-two, and the assumption was made that she was, and always had been, "senile."

The doctors on duty rushed to administer powerful tranquilizers—first Valium and, when that did not help, Haldol—to calm Mrs. Goode so she would not pull out her intravenous tubes and endanger herself. Not for seven hours did anyone think to take a reading on the level of gases in Mrs. Goode's blood, a test that would have been routine in the post-lung surgery work-up of a middle-aged patient with the same symptoms. When this determination finally was made, seven hours after the episode began, Mrs. Goode's system was so sedated by the double dose of tranquilizers that she was in serious danger of going into a coma. The ICU staff had to work frantically to keep her body functions operating before they could begin correcting the problem they had found, belatedly, to have set off her bizarre behavior: an insufficient level of oxygen in the bloodstream, a frequent complication of lung surgery.

"People who are well before surgery don't become disoriented for no reason," Shannon points out. But a severely disoriented eighty-two-year-old patient is considered senile unless proven otherwise—even in the intensive-care unit.

Postoperative complications are not the only reasons the elderly become confused and disoriented in doctors' offices and hospitals. Also at work is fear—fear of pain, fear of illness, fear of death. Like postoperative complications, such fears can arise in patients of any age. But when they occur in the elderly, they are ascribed not to the institutional environment and the alienating feeling of being sick, but to the effects of old age itself—to senility.

In her book *Aging: An Album of People Growing Old*, educator Shura Saul describes a hospitalized man of eighty-seven who, like Mrs. Goode, howls, rages, tears at his tubes and dressings, and is written off as a disoriented senile old man. But Mr. Prince (a pseudonym) is not senile, Saul tells his young physician; he is simply a very difficult patient

213

who has always been unable to deal with stress. He behaved in exactly the same manner when he was fifty-five and underwent a prostate operation, she writes in a chapter called "Open Letter to a Young Doctor," and again at sixty-two when his wife died. When he was seventy-two, he had Ménière's syndrome (intense dizziness and ringing in the ears), and again became disoriented and confused; at eighty and eighty-two, he had heart attacks and behaved in the same bizarre way. But he always managed to recover, holding down a job until he was eighty and taking care of an invalid son until he was eighty-six. "Tell me," Saul implores, "at what point during these past twenty-five years was it correct to attribute his disoriented behavior to his agedness? At sixty-two, when he lost his wife? At seventy, at eighty, at eighty-two—each time during severe physical illness? Yet, each time, he recovered, and continued to function at a level that made younger people, observing him, say, 'Wow, wotta man!' At which point then, Doctor, would it have been accurate to have diagnosed his confusion as inevitable and, possibly, irreversible?

"One cannot know all such things about a patient one is treating," she assures the physician. "That is what makes it so dangerous to apply a stereotype."

The stereotype is applied by many physicians in more routine circumstances as well, as Robert Butler found out during his years as a practicing psychiatrist in Washington, D.C. He often consulted with the other doctors caring for his patients, and was startled to hear a chorus of futility used to describe old people whom Butler had thought to be curable. "Even the most conscientious of physicians [tended] to write off old people as untreatable on the basis of 'age' or 'hardening of the arteries' or 'senility,'" Butler recalls. Often, he says, the doctors volunteered only "pessimistic descriptions of 'organic impairment,' 'irreversibility,' 'limited life expectancy,' and patronizing phrases like 'second childhood,' 'childish,' and 'child-like.' "

The elderly make use of the medical care system more than any other age group in America. Although they compose just under 12 percent of the population, persons over sixty-five account for 25 percent of all prescriptions written, 33 percent of all hospital beds occupied, and 30 percent of all health bills paid. In 1984 the National Center for Health Statistics reported that persons over sixty-five saw physicians at the rate of 6.3 doctor visits per person per year, compared to 4.7 doctor visits per person per year for all age groups.

Old people crowd into doctors' offices and hospital wards for a simple reason: they are more likely to be sick than young people. Most of the chronic illnesses that affect the aged—arthritis, diabetes, hypertension—need a doctor's ongoing care and supervision. The aged are more vulnerable, too, to the major killer diseases, such as heart disease and cancer. But even though old people use the medical care system more, they often are given short shrift by that system. A major study of America's future needs for geriatric manpower, published by the Rand Corporation in 1980, reports that, contrary to conventional wisdom, physicians spend *less* time per person with their elderly patients than they spend with their younger patients.

"The elderly are alleged to take longer to prepare for examination and to comprehend the physician's explanation of diagnosis and treatment," the Rand group, led by Robert Kane of the University of California at Los Angeles, observed. Many physicians use this generalization as a convenient way to write off their elderly patients. To head off the potentially disruptive—and costly—slowness of their older patients, physicians seem to have found a handy answer: they simply refuse to wait. This explains the surprising finding of the Kane group that the older the individual, the *less* time his physician spends with him.

In terms of medical care in nursing homes, physicians have been found to be even more brusque than they are in their own offices. Kane's group pinpointed "a consistent pattern of minimal care" in nursing homes in the United States. "Care given tends to be brief and often superficial, with a conspicuous absence of complete examinations or active attention to therapy. Physician attention appears to be due more to a response to federal regulations than to a commitment to the nursing home patients." Part of medicine's dirty linen, which the profession privately acknowledges but tries to hide from the public, is the degree to which some of the fundamentals of physical examination—breast and pelvic exams in women, and rectal exams in men and women—are "deferred" in patients who are old, especially those who also are institutionalized. Such shortcuts are unforgivable, since these exams are crucial to the diagnosis of several common forms of cancer in their earliest, most treatable stages.

A tendency to brush off the aged as quickly as possible also can lead to the tragic oversight of some physical illnesses that masquerade as "just senility." In the case of the institutionalized aged, approximately 60 percent of whom probably are suffering from Alzheimer's disease, multi-infarct dementia, or some other form of senile dementia, incomplete examinations and hurried physician visits can exaggerate already difficult symptoms of mental infirmity, and can exacerbate the disabilities that come with forgetfulness and confusion. Thus, it is important to look closely at the tendency of the medical profession to rush through its encounters with the aged. Why do so many doctors seem to be in such a hurry?

The answer lies in part in the medical school classroom and the teaching hospital ward. In these training grounds for future physicians, the impression too often relayed is that old patients are more frustrating, more incurable, more expendable than the young. Although more and more medical schools are meeting the challenge of geriatric care with new opportunities in the classroom and the clinic, old biases die hard. Despite the burgeoning of courses in geriatrics, we still see ageism — the deep-seated prejudice against the elderly endemic to Western society — being bred into medical students, interns, and residents during these impressionable years. And at the same time, ignorance about the particular medical, psychological, and social needs of the aged is often allowed, indeed encouraged, to fester.

This chapter will describe the ways in which ignorance and ageism develop in young doctors, and the attempts now being made to bring to physicians-in-training the information they need to treat the aged of tomorrow. Whether they are ready or not, these doctors will find when they enter practice in the 1980s and 1990s that, no matter what specialty they have chosen (with the obvious exception of pediatrics), the majority of their patients will be old.

Medical Schools and the Peter Pan Complex

In a classic experiment conducted in 1968, Donald Spence and his colleagues at the Langley Porter Neuropsychiatric Institute in San Francisco tested the attitudes toward aged patients held by two groups of medical students at the University of California: incoming first-year medical students, with no previous exposure to medical training of any sort, and students entering their fourth year of medical school. Spence found that each group was equally negative in its view of the aged, carrying an image of old people that was "at best an unpleasant one. The old, uniquely amongst age groups, were perceived to possess a political power greater than their soundness of judgment might warrant," Spence reported. "They were perceived as more emotionally ill, disagreeable, inactive, economically burdensome, dependent, dull, socially undesirable, dissatisfied, socially withdrawn, and disruptive of family harmony than youth or adults."

More disturbing to Spence was that "the senior medical students—most of whom will be in active practice within the next five years—after three years of socialization in a profession with an expressed ethic of nondiscrimination and adherence to scientific evaluation of fact rather than unexamined prejudice, did not differ significantly from the freshmen who lacked this experience."

As Spence observed, even though the medical profession expresses a creed of nondiscrimination and of objectivity over prejudice, the message delivered to students on the way to becoming M.D.'s is something quite different. Most of the nation's 127 medical schools teach an ethic of dramatic cure and rapid recovery, heroics in the face of death until death itself is obliterated. Medical professors tend to emphasize in their lectures the diseases for which doctors can prescribe some drug or perform some operation; the chronic illnesses, which are alleviated only through time, patience, and a change in the definition of "cure," are considered too frustrating and too unresponsive to dwell on. "During my first year, when I expressed an interest in geriatrics, I met a lot of resistance to the idea on the part of certain teachers," recalls Richard Shannon, who chaired the task force on aging of the American Medical Student Association (AMSA) while he was a medical student.

"There was kind of the attitude of 'What does a nice young person like you want with something as frustrating and depressing as old people?' "

The first two years of medical school traditionally are devoted to a "core curriculum" of basic biomedical sciences: anatomy, biochemistry, histology, pathology, pharmacology, and physiology. "Until recently, our courses in biochemistry and other basic sciences have always presumed that human life begins at birth and ends at about age fifty," says L. Thompson Bowles, dean for academic affairs at the George Washington University Medical School. Bowles was a prime mover in the effort at GW to introduce more information on aging into these courses. But, like his colleagues at other schools, the best Bowles could do—in deference to scheduling, budgets, and turf disputes—was to offer a patchwork of lectures inserted into already established courses during the first two years. This approach leaves it to the student to tie together the various bits of information into one cohesive impression of senescence.

Despite the generally haphazard approach medical educators take toward teaching geriatrics, medical schools seem to have turned the corner in their move to grant geriatrics a place in the curriculum. In 1976 sixty-three medical schools had no offerings in geriatrics; in 1981 that number was down to thirty-five. But most of the courses available are still superficial, unpopular, and insufficient. "While there has been an overall increase in geriatric educational programs," note Drs. Alan Robbins, Susan Vivell, and John Beck of the University of California at Los Angeles, "The quantity and quality of training . . . are still considerably substandard."

At present, there is still only one free-standing department of geriatrics in the United States: The Gerald and Mary Ellen Ritter Department of Geriatrics and Adult

Development at New York's Mount Sinai Medical Center. But other medical schools have been slow to follow Mount Sinai's lead. For the past twenty years, they have generally resisted efforts on the part of students, government fore- casters, and some faculty members to introduce substantive courses in geriatrics into their curricula. In part, adminis- trators were trying to protect the integrity of their tradi- tional basic science courses, already bombarded by demands from students to make room for courses in community health, behavioral sciences, humanistic medicine, and human sexuality. In part, administrators were responding to a general feeling in the medical community, expounded by groups such as the AMA, that geriatrics does not consti- tute a distinct body of knowledge, and the elderly need no special treatment or medical care simply because they are old. But much of the explanation for medical schools' slug- gishness in adopting courses in geriatrics may lie in what Robert Butler calls their Peter Pan complex.

"There is almost a Peter Pan sense that medicine should be immediately satisfying and not spoiled by situations which defy the doctor's ability to 'make it all better,' " But- ler says. This attitude often is passed on from teacher to student. Having worked hard, indeed single-mindedly, to achieve a coveted place in medical school, many medical students, like their teachers, are drawn to learning about situations in which their skills as physicians are urgently and uniquely needed. Understandably, these students want to swoop down like knights on white horses and, through surgery or drugs, perform miracles—the kind of miracles that rarely are seen on the chronic-care geriatric wards. But even though rapid dramatic cure is all but impossible for the aged, older patients are still challenging, rewarding, and responsive, Butler says. "The medical care of the old is more complex than that of the young, involving many more elements. Inherent in this is a greater challenge to
220

the perceptions and intellect of physicians — if they can avoid the beguilement of 'fast return' medicine."

The hidden message delivered during the first two years of medical school, though, is that fast medicine is the best medicine. And this is the image that impressionable young medical students carry with them when, in their third year, they become junior doctors on the wards of that venerable behemoth, the teaching hospital.

The Hospital Hustle

After the "basic science" years of medical school, when students spend their fourteen-hour days in the library and the lecture hall, most medical training takes place in the teaching hospital. Third-year students don their short white jackets (to distinguish them from interns and residents, whose jackets are longer), hook stethoscopes around their necks, and join the groups of doctors and doctors-in-training who traipse from sickbed to sickbed teaching, learning, and curing. Students are at the bottom of the hospital hierarchy, performing such routine chores as drawing blood and inserting tubes. Just above them are the house-staff officers: interns, in their first year out of medical school, and residents, pursuing two to four additional years of specialty training. At the top of the heap are attending physicians, who hold faculty appointments at the local medical school and also usually have their own private patients in the hospital.

A truism among young doctors is that internship and residency is a time of psychic and physical stress. Almost all physicians-in-training are severely overworked, with on-call schedules that keep them awake up to forty-eight hours running and workweeks that are seldom less than 100 hours long. In such settings, high-quality medical care —

221

the kind learned about in the relatively placid first two years of medical school—can seem a joke, comprehensive diagnostic work-ups can seem an oddity, and life-and-death decisions can be made by young men and women with not enough sleep or training or experience in fact to make them. Medical students, with no patients of their own to follow, are thrown into this environment to sink or swim. Generally, they attach themselves to the interns, and absorb not only information about medical treatment but also subtle messages about attitudes, priorities, and methods necessary to become part of the medical fraternity. One of the first messages thus received is that the fast-paced teaching hospital has little room for old people.

"The hospital is a setting of high tension, and sometimes students and physicians get flip to cope with the incredible tension," says Bowles of GW. This flippancy translates into the casual use of nasty words to describe certain patients. The words available for old patients are the nastiest. The elderly are called crocks, geezers, fogies, snags, neuropaths, rounders, shoppers, crud, and crap. A term recently applied is "gomer," an acronym for "Get Out of My Emergency Room," reserved for the disoriented old persons who seem to show up from nearby nursing homes in the middle of the night. "Gomers are not just dear old people," explains the anti-hero doctor-in-training of *The House of God*, a novel about a year's internship that has become a cult best seller on medical school campuses. "Gomers are human beings who have lost what goes into being human beings. They want to die, and we will not let them. We're cruel to the gomers, by saving them, and they're cruel to us, by fighting tooth and nail against our trying to save them."

After a year of exposure to such attitudes, the intern/narrator of *The House of God* found that his own opinions had been totally turned around. "I had loved old people," he writes. "Now they were no longer old people, they were gomers, and I did not, I could not, love them."

Medical students learn early that "gomers" and "crocks," whose problems are chronic and who will never become fully well, are unvalued in the teaching hospital. They pick up on the message that the best clerkships are the ones where the patients are young and the illnesses exciting — and treatable. Students rotate through six- and twelve-week clerkships during their last two years of medical school, usually spending twelve weeks each in general medicine and general surgery, and six weeks in specialities such as obstetrics/gynecology, pediatrics, psychiatry, ophthalmology, dermatology, gastroenterology, neurology, and endocrinology. In his University of California survey, Donald Spence found that the students coveted the dramatic rotations and deliberately shunned the aged. He asked his first-year and fourth-year students to rank-order a list of six different wards according to their eagerness to train there. For both classes, the responses were identical: first surgery, then pediatrics, then obstetrics, psychiatry, the eye clinic, and, finally, a geriatric ward for the chronically ill. "It may be that the appeal of the first three choices lies in their being characterized by active medical intervention, usually with quickly achieved and satisfying results," Spence surmised. "They offer accomplishment, drama, and cure by virtue of the physician's skill. Psychiatry also provides a field for therapeusis and cure, as does ophthalmology. Apparently all attractions are lacking in a ward for chronically ill old people."

The fact is, though, that many old people brought into the hospital *do* get better — they just do not get better quickly enough to fit conveniently into the medical student's schedule. As a result of their need to taste a little bit of all fields in six-week nibbles, medical students' time

223

frame is severely telescoped. This serves only to confirm their initial feeling that the aged never get well. "With older people very often you have to wait a long time to see any improvement," said physician Patricia Blanchette, founder in 1976 of AMSA's task force on aging. "When you rotate through a ward in six weeks, you don't see much progress no matter how long you stayed on the ward. But if you learn to wait, if you remember that older people with certain diseases take a long time to improve, then you begin to see the value in what you're doing."

One method that has been used successfully to give students perspective on the aged patients' improvements is the videotape. At the Institute for Rehabilitation Medicine at New York University, elderly stroke patients videotaped at monthly intervals allowed students to see for themselves the state they were in before the students came on duty. "For some patients, the progress is incredible," Blanchette said. "The attending [physician] can show the film to medical students and say, 'You saw this patient today. This is what she looked like six months ago!' "

Also useful is the Teaching Nursing Home, a model educational program funded by NIA that allows medical students to do full rotations at nursing homes nearby. These and other educational tools are used so that the student learns to expect not only a different rate of "cure" for the elderly but a different state at which a "cure" is declared. Medical success for an eighty-year-old is quite different from what it is for a thirty-year-old; a good deal more infirmity can be tolerated in the older patient, so long as he or she is able to live a life of optimal functioning and independence. One way that students can learn to adapt what they consider a "decent outcome" to the particular needs of the elderly is to see firsthand the circumstances in which older patients live. "It's good to be right in the long-term care institution," says Shannon, who spent one month working in the chronic-care wing of the Monroe Community Hospital in Rochester, New York. "It makes you pay attention to the quality of life of these people, and to change your goals in therapy. Much of the goal becomes simply functional. . . . Being in the institution, you get an appreciation for the fact that even severely handicapped people have things they enjoy. Even people who can't walk and can't dress themselves get pleasure out of talking or playing cards, and even they have a life that to them is worth maintaining as long as possible." For young, able-bodied medical students who think they would rather die than lose their freedom and mobility, such a discovery can go a long way toward removing the blinders of ageism.

Of course, many nursing home clerkships can be quite devastating, exposing students to unbearable numbers of disoriented, incontinent, incoherent old people confined to beds or geriatric chairs, spending their days howling or staring at the ceiling. At GW, for example, all third-year students are required to spend time in one of four area nursing homes, and those who end up in the most poorly run institutions often come back shattered. "The students are curious, interested, sympathetic," says academic dean Bowles, "but I think they're a little relieved that they won't have to do this work every day for the rest of their lives." Nor does he blame them: "If a student encounters an eighty-five-year-old with organic brain syndrome who is barely coherent, smelly, unpleasant, he doesn't want to go back. It would be the same if that person were a grandparent living in the same house with you—you would avoid going into his room."

For this reason, people in the forefront of the push for geriatric training in medical school have insisted that exposure to old people not be limited to persons in institu-

225

tions. An emphasis on the aged in hospitals or nursing homes skews reality for medical students, since only 5 percent of the elderly are institutionalized at any one time, and another 10 percent, the so-called "frail elderly," are capable of residing in the community with the aid of good social and nursing services. For students to get an accurate picture of the conditions of aged Americans, they must be exposed to some of the more than 22 million old people who lead independent, active lives, lives that permit them to use their minds and bodies in productive ways, to be as fully human as they ever were.

"If medical students never saw a healthy child, but only saw children dying of grave illnesses and living in futile situations, I'm not sure how many of them would want to go into pediatrics," says Robert Butler. The same holds true for the other end of life: Students must see for themselves how challenging, indeed enriching, their older patients can be. Only then will they be able to deliver good medical care to their elderly patients, who, for young doctors entering general medical practice today, make up as much as 40 to 60 percent of a typical patient load. How frustrating it would be, for doctors as well as patients, if physicians were never trained to deal with the special, chronic problems of the old, and had learned only that elderly patients—the majority of their patients—are always sick, always slow-healing, and always impossible to cure. With an attitude like that, how could they help but feel like failures?

❧ 9 ❧

Environment: The "Senility" Regulator

The skeleton of Mary Larkin's pet cat was rotting away in her bedroom when the Washington, D.C., police officers finally came to see what was wrong. The cat had died two or three weeks before, and Mrs. Larkin had wrapped it in sheets and put it in her bed. When the police came, the stench was overwhelming. Mrs. Larkin was taken to St. Elizabeth's Hospital for the mentally ill.

"Mary Elizabeth Larkin, age unknown," reads LaBarbara Bowman's *Washington Post* account of her plight published in February 1980, "squirreled away in a city-owned apartment building, alone, malnourished, confused, depressed by the deaths of those she loved, was, until last week, one of the District of Columbia's estimated 8,000 hidden elderly, the older persons who need help, but have not been found by the city's social service agencies.

"They live alone, cut off in substandard housing, not eating enough food, and suffering from senility, the slow deterioration of the mind that comes with advancing years."

Bowman's off-the-cuff diagnosis of Mary Larkin as "suffering from senility"—a diagnosis offered also by two physicians cited in the article—grows out of the myth of senility", the belief that any older person who is behaving strangely is suffering from the inevitable destruction of brain cells that is the curse of a long life. Such a diagnosis only goes halfway. Yes, the brain changes with age—but the environment is what makes the difference between an individual's ability to compensate for that change, and her need to succumb to it. In providing details of Mary Larkin's surroundings, Bowman's article plants the seeds of a new understanding of the environmental, not merely physiological, causes of the woman's behavior: stresses of a magnitude that would threaten even the healthiest of minds. When those stresses begin acting on the already compromised brain of a very old woman, they can lead to her inability to deal with challenges and situations that had, just weeks before, been manageable.

We saw in chapter 1, and again in chapter 4, that the environment can profoundly influence the behavior of the aged. In this chapter, we will take a closer look at how this happens, and at some steps that can be taken to minimize the adverse effects of environmental stresses. Mary Larkin is a good place to start. The *Post* reports that she has lived alone for four years, since the death of her husband. In those years, her apartment building turned all-black, and Mrs. Larkin, who is white, became afraid to go out even in broad daylight. She was robbed once in her apartment and mugged several times on the street; she became a prisoner in her own neighborhood, feeling frightened even when locked indoors. When she did go out, it was always in the company of Ruth Grimes, a white woman her age who lived around the corner. Without Mrs. Grimes, Mrs. Larkin would not have had the strength or the interest even to go to the grocery store or to prepare meals in her dingy kitchen. Her lack of attention to her food made Mrs. Larkin a prime candidate for malnutrition and dehydration—which, as we have seen, can cause severe behavioral changes in the aged.

For the last two years, Mrs. Larkin has been without electricity, presumably because her bills were not paid. Nighttimes were spent in near-total darkness, relieved only by an occasional candle, while Mary Larkin and her cat sat alone in fear. Without lights, the "twilight confusion" that often affects frailer old people during the night, when visual cues disappear and people retreat into a world of their own, was aggravated. Each night was a struggle for Mrs. Larkin to remember who and where she was. And without electricity for her refrigerator, the notion of fresh milk, eggs, meat, or produce for the old woman was a joke.

The sudden death of Ruth Grimes in early January sent Mary Larkin into a deep depression. When her pet cat died a week or so later, the old woman seemed to crumble. For the first time in her life, she was utterly, profoundly alone. She had gone without eating for a long time when the police finally found Mary Larkin in early February, sitting alone in an apartment without lights, without food, with only the stench of a decaying cat.

Mary Larkin was a victim of many of the environmental stresses know to create senile behavior: malnutrition, dehydration, sensory deprivation, social isolation, depression. It was these stresses, not merely the "slow deterioration of the mind that comes with advancing years," that made the difference between the woman who had functioned, albeit marginally, a few months earlier and the woman who was admitted to St. Elizabeth's Hospital for the mentally ill in

February. The transfer to the mental hospital added one more environmental stress to the picture: the stress of relocation. Suddenly surrounded by strange fixtures and strange people, Mrs. Larkin had trouble remembering where she was. When reporter Bowman asked to see a picture of Mr. Larkin, Mary Larkin, thinking she was still in her apartment, began searching the walls of the hospital corridor for her husband's photograph. "I don't remember where I live," she confessed. "I'm so mixed up. I hate being this way."

Mrs. Larkin's "senility" cannot be separated from the hell she has lived for the last few years. Her story adds weight to a theme we shall explore in this chapter: that the social environment of the aged actually can create senile behavior—or, on the positive side, improve it.

"Many of the psychological difficulties of older persons appear to result from lack of environmental supports, rather than from the aging process per se," wrote the American Psychological Association's Task Force on Aging in a 1971 policy statement. "Inadequate housing, deterioration of older neighborhoods, anti-therapeutic institutions, poorly located services, inadequate transportation, and architectural barriers to mobility may act directly upon the emotional and physical state of any vulnerable individual, old or young."

We all realize that the environment in which we exist can help to shape our behavior. If we feel comfortable in our surroundings, we become gregarious; if it is too dangerous or difficult to get from here to there, we become sluggish. But environmental cues have an even more profound effect on the weak than the strong—and a greater proportion of the very old tend to be weak. Behavioral scientist M. Powell Lawton of the Philadelphia Geriatric Center calls this the Environmental Docility Hypothesis: "As individual competence decreases, the environment assumes increasing importance in determining well-being." We can see this happening in the elderly. Cues about time and place, aids to memory and organization, become more necessary as the brain ages; devices to amplify sights, sounds, even smells become more important as the senses dim. Unfortunately, old people develop a dependence on supportive surroundings at the very stage in life when they have lost the income, friends, and clout needed to obtain them. According to census data published in 1981, 30 percent of the elderly who live alone are poor. Many of them live in deteriorating neighborhoods, both urban and rural; 20 percent of the aged have homes that qualify as "substandard." The effects of these surroundings, as suggested by Corollary One of Lawton's Environmental Docility Hypothesis — "the low-competent are increasingly sensitive to noxious environments" — can be devastating. Surrounded by decay, the old people who are the frailest and the most vulnerable have been known to decay as well.

Corollary Two to Lawton's Environmental Docility Hypothesis is this: "A small environmental improvement may produce a disproportionate amount of improvement in affect or behavior in a low-competent individual." A safe neighborhood versus an unsafe one, accessibility to friends and relatives versus isolation, enough to eat versus unwillingness or inability to prepare meals, enough to do versus boredom — these choices can have an unexpectedly profound effect on whether the aged brain remains functioning to its fullest potential. More so than the other factors in "senility" that we have investigated — stereotyping, medical ageism, physiological changes, genetic influences — the physical environment of the elderly is amenable to change. The trick is to see to it that the environment becomes one that encourages mental and emotional well-being—and this requires money, planning, and influence in policy-making circles, which few old people enjoy.

The Physical Environment

An inhospitable physical environment can do great damage to the elderly, turning small problems into major disabil-ities that may eventually result in senile behavior. Con-sider the widow who cannot manage the four flights of stairs to her apartment; she puts off going to the market and subsists on insufficient food, which in turn produces the confusion and disorientation of malnutrition. Consider the old man who must cross a major intersection to get to his doctor's office, but who knows that the traffic light is timed so that he can never make it across; he may delay seeking medical help for seemingly minor aches and pains until it is too late. Consider the woman who has trouble with the deep steps of city buses, and who has therefore given up the museum outings she used to love; she spends her days alone at home, unable to read because of failing eyesight, feeling a prisoner in a spent body, bitterly allowing her mind, too, to decay.

The modern world is not made for the aged. Elevator doors close too quickly; street signs are too small; lighting in public spaces carries too much glare and too little illu-mination. Old people seem always to be in the way of some-one who is in a hurry. They need time to get their money at the check-out counter, to mount the steps of the bus, to walk across the street, but they are surrounded by people in a rush, muttering, barking, honking at them to get a move on. Experiments conducted on college-age students, similar to the "pre-experiencing age" studies described in chapter 3, show that this slowness cannot be avoided when certain senses have dimmed, and that the slowness itself can lead to emotional and psychological problems in our fast-paced society. One study at the University of Michigan, for example, involved architecture students who donned special distorting eyeglasses, muffling earplugs, and desensitizing fingertip film and then were told to go out and deal with the world they moved in every day. The frustrations of trying to keep in step proved so trying that one student, driven to the verge of depression, was forced to quit the experiment.

But old people cannot quit. They cannot peel off the glasses and suddenly function as efficiently as they used to. This fact of life is especially frustrating for those who still feel as young as ever emotionally, intellectually, spiritually. After all, they have not become different people simply because they have lived a long time. As British gerontologist Alex Comfort describes it, the contradiction they feel between a willing mind and a weak flesh is "like an involuntary change of dress." One ninety-year-old recalls a story he read once—and now understands—about a very old man who woke up each morning with great plans. He would lie in bed and, if it was a fine, sunny day, would think about having his breakfast outdoors, and afterward walking down to the lake for a little fishing. Excited about the prospect of his summer outing, he would begin to hop out of bed. Only then, when his joints started creaking and his heart started thumping, only when his body intruded into his consciousness, would he remember how old he was.

Thus it is for many people trapped in aged bodies. At first, the physical changes of age bring about physical responses—staying at home, moving less agilely and less often, shopping and cooking less—while the mind still fancies itself young. But eventually, these small shifts of activity can lead to a narrowing of horizons and a withdrawal into oneself that can, in turn, lead to forgetfulness, confusion, disorientation. An old person who has trouble going out or moving about the apartment can spend days in the same chair, failing to take medicine (or taking it improperly), neglecting to eat enough, losing track of time, missing the sound of another human voice. What results may be malnutrition, drug mismanagement, or sheer boredom. The already compromised brain grows weaker still, and the old person becomes, like Mary Larkin, a danger to herself and her neighbors.

But this bleak picture need not develop simply because an old person's physical prowess and the physical world around him have changed. Visiting nurse services, Friendly Neighbors clubs, and Meals on Wheels programs can help relieve the social isolation that often sets off a cycle of confusion in the home-bound. Grocery deliveries and housekeeping assistance can help those with relatively minor physical disabilities. And for old people whose biggest problem is forgetfulness—which seems to plague some one-third of those over the age of eighty—environments also can be geared to minimize the disabilities inherent in memory loss, so that homes and neighborhoods become safe places in which to be forgetful.

"We do it for the blind, we do it for the deaf, we do it for the lame—and we can do it for people with memory loss," says Ernest Gruenberg, chairman of the Department of Mental Hygiene at Johns Hopkins University. Gruenberg and other gerontologists advocate a problem-solving approach to environmental support for the forgetful elderly, using tricks and gadgets that can compensate for the mistakes the old person may make. When the memory impairment is mild, as it is for 15 to 20 percent of the very old, the solutions are relatively easy. Gruenberg's favorite nemesis in the homes of forgetful old people is the gas stove. The scene is replayed all too frequently, he says: The old woman leaves a kettle on the stove, forgets about it, and goes to sleep. The water boils over, dousing the flame, and gas fills the house until a neighbor, smelling it, calls the police. Often, the forgetful individual is institutionalized "for her own good." How much better it would be, says Gruenberg, to see the culprit not as the old woman's failing memory but as her antiquated gas stove. "Why not just buy an electric stove?"

Homes could be rearranged in many other simple ways to reduce the potential hazards of mild memory loss. Visual cues in the kitchen could be used for old people who have given up cooking because they forget what goes where; the cues could range from labels on cabinet doors, to color coding of cabinets housing dishes, cans, or spices, to removing doors altogether and allowing the contents to speak for themselves. Charts, lists, and notes can aid immeasurably in helping a forgetful old person through the fog of memory. A diary kept near the medicine chest can help him remember which pills he took when. (So can the daily arrangement of various pills according to when they are to be taken, or the introduction of dated dispensers such as those used for birth control pills.) A note near the nightstand can help him remember to turn off the stove and the television before going to bed. One woman Gruenberg knew was afraid to go shopping alone because she forgot to lock the back door when she went out the front door. But she noticed that she always remembered to turn off the light as she left, because it was right at the front entrance. Her solution: to clip a note to the light pull asking, "Have you locked the back door yet?"

Irons that turn themselves off when left unattended, doors that must be unlocked from the inside so that keys cannot be forgotten (and a place to keep a spare key nearby so the door does not turn into a fire hazard), computerized telephone dials that connect with frequently called numbers by pressing one remembered digit instead of seven—all such gadgets have been or could be developed. If supplied to the forgetful aged, these devices could help them maintain their independence in safety, and could go a long way toward easing the hazard that may be entailed in living with a mild memory loss.

In the 1960s, some fancier schemes for "prosthetic environments" were proposed to help those with moderate to severe memory loss to live on their own. These surroundings were designed not only to help them negotiate the chores of daily life, but actually to help them improve their states of mental alertness and resourcefulness. The notion was that gadgets could provide the cognitive challenges once provided through commerce with the world at large— an interaction now denied these old people due to mental and physical frailty. Based on the belief that social isolation exacerbates mental infirmity, some gerontologists, such as Ogden Lindsley of the Harvard Medical School, proposed the use of mechanical methods to mimic decision-making and remembering tasks that had kept the mind active in earlier years. To get through a doorway or open the refrigerator, for example, the resident could be required to punch out a sequence of keys in the appropriate order. Different sequences could be used to receive a pleasant, sensory-stimulating "reward," such as a tape of a family member's voice or a familiar song. Lindsley proposed that the tapes used in the reward system would be most pleasant for the aged—and therefore most able to elicit a favorable, mind-exercising response—if they were played back at a speed slower than recorded. Some old people, he theorized, may have trouble processing speech at normal speed, just as some children become impatient waiting for normal-paced speech and seem to prefer the double-time talking and singing of records like Alvin and the Chipmunks. "Expanded narrative" recordings, Lindsley said, might work for the aged as effectively as talking records work for the blind— by opening up a world to which they had been denied access because of physiological limitations.

The Institutional Environment

Such "prosthetic environments" have been proposed both for the individual homes of the frail elderly and for nursing homes and other institutions that house large numbers of the severely impaired. But for buttons and tape recorders to work in institutions, many other environmental barriers must first be transcended. As M. Powerll Lawton notes, for the organically impaired elderly the "institutional milieu verges on sensory deprivation"—a condition long known to lead to rapid cognitive decline in even the most healthy individual.

Institutional surroundings are particularly ill-suited to the maintenance of a healthy mental life. In most nursing homes and other long-term care facilities, all the corridors look alike, all the meals taste alike, all the days feel alike. The residents have little sense of time, little to do from one day to the next. They make few decisions, go nowhere, and are rarely encouraged to think and act for themselves.

Such deficiencies are usually not the doing of heartless, greedy nursing home administrators—although horror stories about profiteering in the industry certainly exist— but are usually simply a function of life in an institution, where rules are made and kept automatically and unimaginatively. Lawton, on the basis of his experience at the

Philadelphia Geriatric Center, points out that even severely impaired old men and women can be helped through subtle changes in their environment that would please anybody: more color, more graphics, more variety of furniture in the decor. He says residents could be aided in their cognitive responses if the ubiquitous "dayroom" were divided into easily differentiated subspaces for reading, playing games, or watching television. At the very least, Lawton says, staff members should encourage the residents, especially those most impaired, to change chairs or move from one area to another at a specified time of day. Otherwise, hours blend into each other, and one day of the week looks and feels exactly like the next. Such monotony is sure to hasten the rate of mental deterioration.

Lawton's Environmental Docility Hypothesis—that the lower an individual's level of competence, the more he or she is affected, adversely or positively, by the environment—is demonstrated most dramatically in the institutional setting. One study of mobility patterns among old people in eight British nursing homes revealed that the most impaired patients were most likely to stay in their rooms or, if they did emerge, to occupy the least desirable seats in the public spaces. Conversation with other confused patients was rare, and mixing with the mentally intact almost unheard of. Conversely, another study showed that apparently small changes in the surroundings, in this case rearranging the dayroom furniture from a chairs-around-the-perimeter configuration to friendlier clusterings of tables and chairs, can indeed change the social behavior of even the most impaired residents. Although the essential downward progression of their mental disabilities was not halted by such changes, their ability to think, or at least to communicate, was improved, as was their quality of life, by a simple reshuffling of some furniture. (Interestingly, the most difficult aspect of this experiment was preventing the patients and staff from rearranging the furniture each day back to the perimeter arrangement they were accustomed to.)

Other seemingly minor changes have also been shown to have big impacts on nursing home residents. A daily wine break at 3:00 P.M. was found in one nursing home to lead to a "social club" camaraderie among many residents who previously had not communicated at all. The chance to make a few decisions—whether and when to receive visitors, which plants to have in their rooms—helped residents at another home maintain both physical and psychological health. But according to Lawton, while such studies are enlightening, the results are quite beside the point. Even if conviviality and mood were *not* shown to improve after surroundings were upgraded, the elderly in nursing homes would still have "inalienable environmental rights" that must be respected. For too long, he says, we have tolerated ugly, unsafe, dirty, impersonal surroundings in these institutions, and have excused them "because they presumably are not salient to the organic brain syndrome patient. Why should we have to prove that this assertion is false?" The assumption should be that mentally impaired old people, as much as anyone else, deserve (and appreciate) surroundings that are as attractive as they can be within the constraints of money, space, and function.

Lawton has had a chance to put these ideas into practice at the Philadelphia Geriatric Center (PGC). The long-term-care wing at PGC for "organic brain syndrome" patients was designed to combine aesthetics with function in a manner that at the time was unique to nursing home care. The most dramatic innovation in the new wing is its scrapping of the traditional institutional corridor in favor of a huge, brightly lit "central space" measuring 40 by 100 feet.

"The long hallway has for years been recognized as contributing to the debasing environment of many institutions, and to disorientation," Lawton notes. "Detail disappears quickly in perspective; at best one can perceive a couple of—usually identical—room doors beyond the point where one is standing." In the PGC wing, patients' rooms, each with a different, bright color scheme that extends to the doorjamb, are arranged around three sides of the central space, most of which is used as "an informal social area, articulated by easily movable groupings of furniture." A plant-filled gazebo serves as a visual focal point at one end of the space, and behind the gazebo is an area for crafts, games, and therapeutic activities. At the other end of the central space is a clearly demarcated dining area, the sight of which serves as a clue to time of day. The nurses' station projects into the center of the activity. All spaces are large enough easily to accommodate wheelchairs and walkers, thus encouraging independent mobility, and the central space is supplied with cues to time and place, such as a prominent clock and a "reality orientation board" naming the date, the weather, the next meal, and the next holiday.

The wing's design incorporates many of the devices suggested for use at the noninstitutional level. The open treatment area, says Lawton, "is intended to diminish the effects of disorientation and memory loss by giving residents an almost complete view of all areas from anywhere in the space." Similarly, doors can be opened only when two buttons are pressed simultaneously," a task that is impossible for the impaired wanderer to master," thus making further restraints on such residents unnecessary.

But Marimekko fabric wall hangings and Scandinavian-design chairs cannot hide the fact that the residents of this wing are mentally impaired, most of them suffering from Alzheimer's disease. And, for all the potted plants and natural-wood floors, the residents' intellectual functioning and ability to care for themselves seem to decline as rapidly here as they would have on a traditional, pea-green-colored ward. There is a difference in the new wing, though: Lawton says the residents here socialize more, participate more in "enriching activity," and show more interest in their surroundings. Family members and friends visit more often than they did on the older ward, and staff members prefer the new environment, making for greater affability all around.

For all that institutional environments can be improved, though, most old people probably would best be served if they could be kept out of institutions altogether. Often, one annoying habit or particular quirk is what leads an old person or the family to consider institutionalization—a tendency to wander, incontinence, continual near-misses with the kettle on the gas stove. If a system existed through which residents could be admitted to nursing homes on a short-term basis, suggests Gruenberg of Johns Hopkins, perhaps this single habit could be sufficiently curbed to allow the individual to return, possibly with new environmental supports, to independent living.

This will, of course, require a major rethinking on the part of relatives of the aged, who now assume that once such habits begin, they will last a lifetime. The decision to institutionalize a loved one, no matter how good the nursing home, is a heart-wrenching one, made only after the family has tried every other means to help the old person function in the community. If suddenly the institution were to release him, saying he has been trained to use the bathroom properly, or to find his way home, or to sleep more regular hours, the family would have to undo the private grieving that had preceded the decision to institutionalize in the first place.

If such a scheme of short-term institutionalization were to work, there must also be a place to which the old person could return to live in comfort and safety. Without the supportive environment necessary to compensate for mild memory loss, plans for independence for the forgetful aged are just idle talk. Other Western countries, particularly those in Scandinavia, have experimented with possible solutions to this problem, testing innovative housing arrangements that serve those aged persons who are too impaired to live wholly on their own but not impaired enough to move into nursing homes. One successful approach is called "congregate housing," where the elderly live in their own high-rise apartments but have accessible in the same building a range of services such as housekeeping, shopping, doctors' offices, and sometimes even common dining rooms. In this country, similar arrangements have been tried on a more informal basis, and some groups are experimenting with ad hoc "communes" for the elderly, with private bedrooms (occasionally with their own baths and kitchenettes) and communal areas for socializing, cooking, and eating.

The environment is a factor in mental functioning at all stages of life, but most forcefully, it seems, in old age. In a deprived environment, both brain cells and idiosyncratic compensatory tricks wither away, leaving an aged individual alone in a harsh world that moves by too quickly, and that defines the old person's slowness and confusion as "senility." Once categorized as senile, the elderly are passed off to isolated environments, both in institutions and in the community, that further deprive them of an opportunity to remain alert and functioning.

But the silver lining in this story is that, while old people are particularly vulnerable to environmental stresses, they are also particularly responsive to environmental supports. Old brains are remarkably pliable, capable of springing back to life—in terms of both revived personalities and actual regenerated brain cells—if conditions are ripe. This fact adds a poignant urgency to the growing cry that the elderly deserve an honored place in Western society. To deny them that place is to deny them the opportunity not only to maintain their mental functioning but also to grow.

•*10*•

A Look to the Future

This book's message is essentially optimistic: Most old people do not "go senile" no matter how long they live. But while our findings about anatomical and functional brain aging are cheering, they have been tempered by the harsh effects of other kinds of aging—sociological and psychological. The biological changes encountered over time generally are rather benign and easily transcended, but the social and cultural constraints under which those changes occur can turn the picture from one of a gentle downward slope into an avalanche.

Physically, the brain becomes smaller, lighter, and looser with age. Billions of brain cells, or neurons, have died, and the cells that remain often have lost the branch-like extensions, called dendrites, needed to communicate with neighboring cells. Pieces of debris accumulate in the spaces between and within cells, including the yellowish "age pigment" known as lipofuscin, masses of degenerating cellular matter called neuritic plaques, and twisted arrangements of neuronal bits called neurofibrillary tangles. These excess components, and the proliferation of tiny brain cells known as glial cells, tend to plug up the works in the aged brain, already at a disadvantage due to the loss of neurons.

The old brain is characterized too by a sharp reduction in neurotransmitters. Neurotransmitters, the ferrymen of the brain's communication system, are chemicals released by neurons to aid in the transfer of specific signals between specific brain cells. The transmitter acetylcholine is thought to have a major role in the process of memory — and, significantly, it has been shown to decrease by as much as 70 percent in the healthy aged brain. Also reduced are such essential neurotransmitters as dopamine, epinephrine, norepinephrine, and GABA (gamma-amino-butyric acid).

The anatomical changes that have been documented in the brains of healthy old people don't always lead to predictable functional changes. The great majority of the elderly are able to compensate for their physical losses, maintaining the same mental skills they had throughout life. Only two functions show almost universal, though usually mild, decline: speed of response and memory. Social factors explain some of these changes. Old people generally have not received the education needed to conceptualize facts in such a way that they can be recalled easily to mind, and they usually aren't as schooled in test taking, or as motivated to perform well on those tests, as are the younger individuals with whom their scores are unfavorably compared. With intellectual skills for which speed is not a relevant factor, such as vocabulary, many persons actually improve with age. And when old people are properly trained to perform on tests of "fluid," or abstract, intelligence, their test scores show that time is not the great stealer we used to think it was.

Memory, like speed of thought, does indeed seem to slip over the years, but that need not be a debilitating problem either. Psychologists distinguish between the benign and malignant forms of memory loss, and point out that fear, tension, and social pressure can help nudge the benign toward the malignant. Benign forgetfulness is when you misplace your glasses; malignant forgetfulness is when you forget you ever had glasses. When they are not paralyzed with the expectation that every memory lapse brings them one step closer to "senility," old people have proven quite resourceful in finding ways around those benign lapses — writing notes, leaving clues, using mnemonic devices, or simply ignoring the forgotten name or place and allowing it to reemerge, unnoticed, a few minutes or even a few hours later.

Complaints about forgetfulness in the elderly are often associated not with objective memory loss, but with depression. Depressed persons tend to turn to the available stereotype for a definition of themselves, and depressed old persons are likely to think of themselves as worthless, mindless, senile. Depression at any age can masquerade as a host of physical illnesses, from bronchitis to heart attack; in the elderly, it is the most common cause of the syndrome called "pseudosenility."

Pseudosenility occurs when a doctor is confronted with an elderly patient complaining of confusion, disorientation, and memory loss, and diagnoses the patient as senile. In perhaps as many as one out of five cases, that diagnosis is dead wrong; The patient is suffering not from a chronic, irreversible condition but from a physical illness that may be 100 percent treatable. Because of the brain changes that occur with age, most healthy elderly persons are able to remain alert and functioning only through a complex set of compensatory mechanisms. When the system is stressed by any sort of physical complaint, ranging from a bad cold or anemia to a heart attack or appendicitis, those mechanisms break down, and the brain—the weakest link—is the first place to show signs of strain. As many as 100 physical disorders have been identified that in the elderly produce none of the classic symptoms seen in middle age. Their most typical manifestations in the elderly are confusion, disorientation, and memory loss. To a family member or a physician who is less than alert, these symptoms look very much like "senility," and the elderly patient may miss out on medical treatment that could have reversed the underlying condition.

In some cases, though, the senile symptoms are caused not by physical illness, nor by drug intoxication—another common cause of pseudosenility—but by a real disease affecting the brain itself. The confusion, disorientation, and memory loss may be due to one of several irreversible disorders, such as multi-infarct dementia (once mistakenly called "hardening of the arteries of the brain"), Korsakoff's psychosis, Creutzfeld-Jakob disease, or the dementias associated with Parkinson's disease or Huntington's chorea. But in more than half the cases, the symptoms are caused by Alzheimer's disease, a neurological disorder that at present is progressive and incurable.

Alzheimer's disease, first described in 1906 by the German pathologist Alois Alzheimer, is thought to affect 2 to 3 million Americans in middle and old age, and has been ranked as the nation's fourth or fifth leading killer. Diagnosis of the disease cannot be made with conviction until the patient dies, when a brain autopsy reveals characteristic changes. In the brains of persons with Alzheimer's disease, the neuritic plaques and neurofibrillary tangles found to some small degree in most old persons have proliferated wildly, especially in the essential brain regions of the cerebral cortex and hippocampus, regions responsible for thought and memory. The plaques and tangles have been directly correlated with the intellectual decline observed in Alzheimer's patients: the more plaques and tangles, the greater the cognitive loss is.

Neurologists are now investigating other characteristics of Alzheimer's brains in hopes of someday finding its cause — and, ultimately, a treatment or even a means of preventing it. Among the intriguing findings is that the neurotransmitter acetylcholine, which is reduced by as much as 70 percent in the brains of normal old people, declines to less than 10 percent of its highest level in persons with Alzheimer's disease. In addition, the concentration of aluminum in Alzheimer's brains has been found to be three times normal — a discovery that is especially intriguing in light of the fact that aluminum has been implicated as a cause of other forms of dementia, such as the profound disorientation sometimes associated with long-term dialysis therapy for kidney patients. Scientists are also investigating the theory that Alzheimer's disease is caused by a slow virus, an infectious agent that can remain dormant for years and that flares up and begins to cause symptoms when the individual's internal or external environment changes. And they are studying family trees and the relationship between Alzheimer's and certain genetic diseases to try to determine how much of Alzheimer's disease is carried on the genes. At present, they believe that Alzheimer's disease is not inherited in the same way that sickle-cell anemia, for example, is inherited, but rather that the tendency to develop Alzheimer's, like the tendency to develop breast cancer or heart disease, may run in families.

Because it threatens to rob people of their most precious asset—their personalities, their very concepts of themselves—Alzheimer's disease sends its victims, and their families, rushing after any promise of a cure. Doctors today can offer no such promises. Therefore, Alzheimer's patients are vulnerable to the anti-senility claims of proponents of a variety of over-the-counter preparations, such as choline, lecithin, nicotinic acid, vitamin E, RNA, and (available only in Nevada) Gerovital H-3. Not only Alzheimer's patients, but all old people worried about whether a "senile" future awaits them, seem willing to try anything that promises them a better memory and a better mind.

Most of these self-help medications have proved disappointing, as have the prescription drugs scientists have tested in controlled clinical studies: Hydergine, L-dopa, centrophenoxine, and Piracetam. Until researchers find the cause of Alzheimer's disease, and the underlying mechanism for the degeneration that often accompanies aging, doctors will be left with shot-in-the-dark attempts at relieving the symptoms when mental infirmity strikes.

In this context, physicians become counselors rather than curers, since there is little they can do for patients suffering the disabilities of old age. The best they can offer is to help these patients maintain those mental functions that remain. This requires a "holistic" approach to the patient, an openness to seeing physical problems in terms of the social and psychological climate, an ability to coordinate medical care with support from other kinds of therapists, and a willingness to stop short of heroic "cures" and to measure success in the patient's terms. Such attitudes rarely are transmitted in medical schools, where students learn to revere the quick, dramatic cure of the prescription pad or the surgeon's knife. In most medical schools today, old patients do not fit the convenient medical model of diagnosis, prognosis, treatment, and cure. They are therefore perceived as irritating reminders of doctors' inability to "make everything all better," and they are, in general, mistreated or ignored.

The mood is changing, however, as more medical students come to realize that, no matter what specialty they choose (except for pediatrics and obstetrics), the majority of their patients will be old. Encouraged by a handful of leaders in the field of geriatrics, medical students have been pushing for the introduction of more geriatrics courses in their schools. The schools, notoriously slow to change their curricula, are at last beginning to respond. About two-thirds of the nation's 127 medical schools now include some course work in geriatrics—the content, quality, and popularity of which vary widely—and the rest are expected to follow in the next ten or fifteen years.

Such courses contain, at a minimum, the body of medical knowledge unique to older patients—the age-related changes in drug metabolism, for example, that make old people particularly vulnerable to overmedication and to the adverse effects of drug-drug interactions. In addition, good courses in geriatrics will include a healthy dose of medical sociology, describing ways in which the old person's environment can affect health and mental functioning. As the Environmental Docility Hypothesis of gerontologist M. Powell Lawton states, the less competent the individual, the more important the environment becomes in shaping his or her well-being.

The environment of many old people—especially the thousands who are poor and living in deteriorating neighborhoods—is enough to push them over the fine line separating compensation from "senility." But the environment also can be what pulls those same people back to healthy functioning. With proper environmental supports, many "senile" people are able to live independent lives in the community, or to live in institutions without becoming totally dependent and vegetative. Such support includes visual and tactile reminders of what goes where and what is done when, help with chores and routines that the individual is unable to handle, and surroundings that are attractive, simple, and easily negotiated alone. "Prosthetic environments" have been suggested for use in nursing homes and other institutions, and they can be adapted to the homes of the mentally frail elderly in order to help them maintain their ability to think, reason, and make decisions for themselves.

Since surroundings are so important in determining the course of disorders such as Alzheimer's disease—as well as the ultimate resolution of the milder mental changes of old age—friends and relatives of the aged, and the old people themselves, are more important than are health professionals in determining whether the mental life of the aged will be empty or full. Their attitudes and their expectations give form and meaning to the slips and lapses that accompany healthy old age, and can minimize the disabilities that are inevitably a part of progressive diseases like Alzheimer's.

What Attitude Fits?

Your attitude after reading this book will be formed in part from your reason for reading it in the first place. You may be young or middle-aged and curious (or worried) about the years ahead. You may be old and, while still healthy and functioning, concerned about the changes you've already observed in your mental agility. You may love someone who is old, and may wonder why he or she is not performing up to par. In each case, the lessons learned from the preceding nine chapters can help you to chip away at your belief in the myth of senility, and to carve out instead a comfortable niche for your image of mental life in old age, an image that has room for healthy, engaged, intelligent men and women.

If you are middle-aged, the essential message of our study is this: Keep active. Involvement in challenges outside yourself will keep your mind busy and alert. Keep healthy, too; physical health is the most important determinant of mental health in old age. And, since "senility" can be a self-fulfilling prophecy that makes people unwittingly turn themselves into the creatures they expect to become, learn to expect to stay well.

If you're in your middle years, you can also take a cue from the late anthropologist Margaret Mead, who remained a major figure in American thought until her death at age seventy-eight in 1979. "Change all your doctors, opticians, and dentists when you reach fifty," she said in a 1977 interview. "You start out when you are young with everybody who looks after you older than you are. When you get to be fifty, most of these people are sixty-five or older. Change them all and get young ones. Then, as you grow older, you'll have people who are still alive and active taking care of you. You won't be desolate because every one of your doctors is dead." The same can be said for your friends, and for the same reason. If all your friends are from your generation, and you are lucky enough to live a long time, your old age is likely to be clouded with feelings of loneliness and abandonment as your dear friends die. But if you cultivate friendships with younger people during your middle age, you will continue to have a new store of friends who are still alive when you're old, friends who can still engage you in a world outside yourself.

253

If you are old and healthy, don't let your occasional lapses of memory scare you. Forgetfulness plagues us all, at any age, and simply plagues us more often as we age. Your thinking and remembering will slow down a little, but the slowing is harmless so long as you can keep it in perspective. Again, expectations are the key: If you expect to become more forgetful—which you will—your memory loss won't take you by surprise, and you can learn to use tricks to compensate for it. If you expect to "go senile"—which, odds are, you won't—you may indeed turn those occasional lapses into a debilitating problem for which you cannot compensate. Remember that there is a difference between benign forgetfulness and malignant forgetfulness, and an expectation of profound memory loss can nudge the one toward the other.

Invent ways to keep your mind in gear. Set up challenges for yourself, even if they seem difficult at first—accept new assignments, read new books, meet new people, learn new skills. And don't be too stubborn, or too vain, to seek help when help is needed, whether it be with shopping or housekeeping or going to the doctor or balancing the checkbook. Your independence need not be threatened—indeed, it may be preserved—by an intelligent, well-reasoned admission of your dependence.

These guidelines, of course, should not be taken too literally. There are some people who would like nothing better in their old age than to curl up and do nothing. As California psychologist Richard Kalish says, the prevalent "geriactivist model" of "successful" aging overlooks these people. "Something is assumed to be wrong with older people who wish to sit around and talk with elderly friends," he says, "who wish to stay at home and read, who thoroughly enjoy television, who for whatever reason prefer their world to be comfortable, comforting and manageable rather than stimulating, challenging and risky." If that is your style, don't apologize for it. You've waited a long time for the leisure offered by retirement and grown children so you can spend your days quietly.

By the same token, be sure that you are not retreating to the "comfortable, comforting and manageable" as a way to escape the frustration brought about by the "stimulating, challenging and risky." Newness always brings with it some measure of failure and disappointment; these sentiments are not the sole province of the old. If you remember that your struggle with a new book or a new skill is the result of your unfamiliarity with it, not your age, perhaps the frustrations will be easier to manage.

If your loved one is old and becoming impaired, try to treat him or her as you always did. Include her (let's say it's your mother) in family decisions, listen to her stories and her advice, wait out her occasional memory lapses with patience, not fear and worry. If the changes you observe seem to be the milder age-related changes you've read about—a slowing down in thought, a greater tendency to forget—talk about them with your mother, and reassure her that she's unlikely to become seriously disabled by these losses, of which she is no doubt aware. Walk a fine line between over- and under-expectations: reduce your demands on your loved one (frustrating her unnecessarily will only make matters worse), but don't shut her out, and above all don't do things for her that she can still do herself.

If you observe significant changes in your relative's mental capacities—if, for instance, your husband suddenly seems unable to reason or think logically, or to say where he is, or what day it is—take him to a doctor. Insist on a thorough medical exam—and a real diagnosis. A physician who dismisses the case with a quick label of "Alzheimer's disease," "senile dementia," or some other non-diagnosis is telling you nothing. Make sure the doctor carefully rules out drug intoxication, depression, and the many treatable medical conditions that can account for sudden "senility." Do not accept a diagnosis of an irreversible syndrome until the doctor has done so.

If, after thorough testing, the diagnosis *is* irreversible Alzheimer's disease, don't despair. "Irreversible is not synonymous with deteriorating," notes Gene Cohen of the National Institute of Mental Health. Your parent or spouse may have years of good functioning ahead, with support from you to get over the rough spots. Help your loved one maintain independence for as long as possible, try to keep him or her active in as many pursuits as feasible, and surround him or her with as many familiar people, places, and routines as you can.

Perhaps the most difficult thing to remember, in watching a loved one with Alzheimer's disease, is that even though many skills might be lost, many still remain. Long after your relative—say, in this case, your wife—has forgotten her way home, she may still be capable of singing along to old tunes on the radio. Long after she has lost the ability to make sense of a movie or a television show, she may still be able to listen to, understand, and discuss the news. Learn what she still can do, and allow her to do it.

The course of Alzheimer's disease is quite idiosyncratic, but most patients eventually need some sort of institutional care in the very latest stages. At this point, some patients lose their ability to control their urinary and bowel functions, and may require round-the-clock nursing care and, in some cases, high-technology life support. Depending on the family situation, institutionalization may be necessary even before this stage. It may prove impossible to care at home for an old man or woman who wanders out of the house at night and can't find the way home, or who flies off into inexplicable tantrums, or who must be left alone all day and has a habit of overflowing the bathtub or throwing lit matches onto the floor. If this is your situation, no one will be served if you martyr yourself and your family for the sake of a loved one with Alzheimer's disease. A nursing home or some other facility is the only solution, and it is a solution that you should approach, if possible, with a minimum of guilt.

In the future, perhaps the choices about treatment for patients with Alzheimer's disease will be less dismal. Scientists are bursting with ideas about possible causes for Alzheimer's and one of the many research routes they are now taking is likely to bear fruit in the next ten or fifteen years. They are investigating theories ranging from aluminum intoxication to slow virus infection, from genetic markers to chromosomal abnormalities, from immune disorders to neurotransmitter deficiencies. "It is entirely possible that none of [these] theories will turn out to be correct," observes Robert Butler of Mount Sinai Medical Center at New York. "But when I entered this field thirty years ago, there were no viable theories regarding the causes of Alzheimer's disease. Mental impairment was simply accepted as an unavoidable concomitant of the aging process."

But scientific opportunity alone does not always warrant optimism about the future course of research on a particular disease. All the good ideas in the world are worthless if researchers cannot find grant money with which to pursue those leads. Fortunately, in the case of Alzheimer's disease, scientific interest and political (read: fiscal) interest are peaking simultaneously. In the fickle world of biomedical research priorities, old people have become the constituency of the decade, and Alzheimer's seems to be the disease of the moment.

257

Researching the Future

To understand why this is reason for cheer, one first must understand the vagaries of biomedical research funding. The first point to remember is that American scientists depend almost exclusively on government grants to support their work. The allocation of these grants, for which competition is fierce, is determined not only by the quality of the experiment but also by the popularity of the topic on Capitol Hill and in the federal bureaucracy. The government does not support science out of the goodness of its collective heart, nor out of a driving curiosity to find out how the world works. When it spends millions on a particular study, it expects someday to be able to exhibit discoveries that will have an impact on the daily lives of a grateful public. Like any other big enterprise, it wants a return on its investment.

Thus, a courtly mazurka is danced by members of congress, federal officials, and scientists as they go about setting the national research agenda. Throughout the dance, an ear is cocked to hear the rumblings of the American electorate, to learn what diseases are killing, maiming, and frightening the greatest number. Until recently, the loudest voices heard were those concerned with cancer, so the dance card of cancer researchers was regularly filled to overflowing while scientists in gerontology, neuroscience, and other quieter fields were turned into wallflowers. But in the past few years, since the war on cancer of the early 1970s was officially de-escalated, studies of aging, and especially of the dementias of aging, have been thrown into the limelight. The voices of an ever-growing minority of Americans, the elderly, are finally being heard.

The federal biomedical research establishment is dominated by the National Institutes of Health (NIH), a $5 billion branch of the Department of Health and Human Services. Congress determines the size and scope of the NIH budget, making it a highly political document that reflects in large part the relative stridency of various constituency groups. When the National Institute on Aging (NIA) was formed in 1974, joining ten other institutes on the sprawling NIH "campus" in a suburb of Washington, D.C., it reflected Congress's appreciation of the growing clout of the elderly. At the time, persons over sixty-five represented 15 percent of eligible voters in the United States, and they participated in elections more than almost any other age group: 90 percent were registered to vote, and 65 percent voted regularly. Since then, powerful lobbying groups—from the 18-million-strong American Association of Retired Persons to the militant Gray Panthers—have captured the attention of politicians and the media alike, and NIA has continued to reap the windfall. Since its founding, NIA's budget has increased nearly nine-fold, from $16 million to more than $140 million, at a time when the overall budget for NIH has barely kept up with inflation.

The scientists competing for a slice of this still-growing NIA pie have taken a cue from cancer researchers, who managed to help engineer their own windfall during the war on cancer of the 1970s. Gerontologists are finally learning the meaning of the word "lobby." A prime example of their new political sophistication was the formation in 1979 of the Alzheimer's Disease and Related Disorders Association, a national umbrella group formed to unite into one loud voice the small self-help groups that were forming across the country. In that same year, Alzheimer's disease was designated one of the Department of Health and Human Services' top ten research priorities for the 1980s, and the NIA inaugurated two new programs to follow it up: a Neurosciences Program at the institute's

Gerontology Research Center in Baltimore and a Social and Behavioral Research Program at its Bethesda, Maryland, headquarters.

The rising political fortunes of gerontological research are indeed cause for cheer—but the optimism must be tempered somewhat by the reminder that, despite the comparable popularity of cancer research in the 1970s, a cure for cancer still eludes us. As scientists are quick to tell an impatient Congress and a disappointed public, scientific breakthroughs cannot be bought. A technological "fix" for Alzheimer's disease and some of the other mental changes of age—a vaccine, a pill, a miraculous operation— probably does not wait in the wings. For many years to come, the best prescription for a mentally healthy old age will probably remain what it is today: patience, love, and an enlightened awareness that most old folks need never go senile.

Notes

1. THE MYTH OF SENILITY

The quote from Robert Butler, and the survey and figures to back it up, are taken from an interview on Dec. 28, 1977. The description of the NIMH personality studies he was involved with in the 1950s is from another interview, July 8, 1978.

Marian Cleeves Diamond's experiment on enriched and deprived environments is described in her article "The aging brain: some enlightening and optimistic results." *American Scientist*, vol. 66, Jan.–Feb. 1978, pp. 66–71.

Claude Oster describes the "cephalopedal" reflex in "Sensory deprivation in geriatric patients," *Journal of the American Geriatrics Society*, vol. 24, no. 19, 1976, pp. 461–64.

The NIMH aging study was written up as *Human Aging I: A Biological and Behavioral Study,*Washington, D.C.: U.S. Government Printing Office, 1974. Authors are James E. Birren, Robert N. Butler, Samuel W. Greenhouse, Seymour Perlin, Louis Sokoloff, and Marian R. Yarrow. A second report, *Human Aging II: An Eleven-Year Followup Biomedical and Behavioral Study*, Washington, D.C.: U. S. Government Printing Office, 1976, was compiled by S. Granick and R. D. Patterson. A similar longitudinal study of healthy aging was described in another two-volume work, *Normal Aging*, published in 1965 (vol. I) and 1974 (vol. II) by Duke Univerity Press, Durham, N.C., and edited by Erdman Palmore.

Information from Thomas Kalchthaler was gathered during an interview on Dec. 22, 1977.

John Blass's estimates of the prevalence of different types of senile dementia were reproduced graphically in "A Slow Death of the Mind" by Matt Clark et al., *Newsweek*, Dec. 3, 1984, p. 59.

Robert Katzman determined Alzheimer's disease to be the nation's fourth or fifth leading killer in "The prevalence and malignancy of Alzheimer's disease: A major killer," *Archives of Neurology*, vol. 33, no. 4, 1976, pp. 217–18.

The hereditability of Alzheimer's disease is the topic of "Alzheimer's: New Genetic Evidence" by Sandy Rovner, *The Washington Post*, April 24, 1985, Health section p. 15.

The relationship between brain lesions and degree of dementia is best described by Garry Blessed, Bernard E. Tomlinson, and Martin Roth in, "The association between quantitative measures of dementia and senile change in the cerebral grey matter of elderly subjects," *British Journal of Psychiatry*, vol. 114, 1968, pp. 797–811.

2. BRAIN CHANGES WITH AGE: FORM VS. FUNCTION

Much of the information in this chapter is derived from Robert Terry's chapter, "Physical changes of the aging brain," in *"The Biology of Aging*, John A. Behnke, Caleb E. Finch, and Gairdner B. Moment (eds.), New York: Plenum Press, 1978, pp. 205–20.

Carl Eisdorfer's comment was made in an interview on May 24, 1979.

Harold Brody describes his work on cell counts in his chapter, "Cell counts in cerebral cortex and brainstem," in *Alzheimer's Disease: Senile Dementia and Related Disorders*, Robert Katzman, Robert D. Terry, and Katherine L. Bick (eds.), New York: Raven Press, 1978, pp. 345–51. He first published his findings in "Organization of cerebral cortex. III. A study of aging in the human cerebral cortex," *Journal of Comparative Neurology*, vol. 102, 1955, pp. 511–56.

The Scheibels' work is described in "Progressive dendritic changes in the aging human limbic system," by Madge E. Scheibel, Robert D. Lindsay, Uwamie Tomiyasu, and Arnold B. Scheibel, *Experimental Neurology*, vol. 53, 1976, pp. 420–30. Paul Coleman's work appears in "Morphology of the aging central nervous system: Not all downhill" (with Christine A. Curcio and Stephen J. Buell), *The Aging Motor System*, J. A. Morhmer, F. J. Pirozzolo, G. S. Maletta (eds.) New York: Praeger, 1982, pp. 7–35.

Christian de Duve's comment was made in "Cells age: Are lysosomes among the villains?" in *Aging into the 21st Century: Middle-Agers Today*, Lissy F. Jarvik (ed.), New York: Gardner Press, 1978, p. 25.

Kalidas Nandy's comment comes from "Morphological changes in the aging brain," in *Senile Dementia: A Biomedical Approach*, Kalidas Nandy (ed.), New York and Amsterdam: Elsevier/North-Holland Biomedical Press, 1978, pp. 19–32.

Robert Terry's comments on lipofuscin accumulation were made in his chapter in *The Biology of Aging*, cited above.

The Swiss research on blood vessel changes is described in "Alterations of morphological and neurochemical parameters of the brain due to normal aging," by W. Meier-Ruge, O. Hunziker, P. Iwangoff, K. Reichlmeier, and P. Sandoz, in Nandy's *Senile Dementia,* cited above.

Holger Hyden's work with RNA in glial cells is described by Antonia Vernadakis in "Neuronal-glial interactions during development and aging," in *Biology of Aging and Development*, G. Jeanette Thorbecke (ed.), New York and London: Plenum Press, 1975, p. 176.

The "neural noise" hypothesis is described by A. T. Welford, "On changes of performance with age," *Lancet*, Feb. 17, 1962, pp. 335–39. Excerpts of this article appear in *Human Ageing*, Sheila M. Chown (ed.), Baltimore: Penguin Books, 1972, pp. 95–99.

David Drachman describes his work in "Human memory and the cholinergic system: A relationship to aging?" (with Janet Leavitt), *Archives of Neurology,* vol. 30, Feb. 1974, pp. 113–21.

Robert Terry mentions the neurotransmitter changes of age in his chapter in *The Biology of Aging*, cited above. Peter Davies's comments are from an interview on Jan. 16, 1981.

Lissy Jarvik's comment on MAO was made in an interview on May 24, 1979.

Old people's ability to metabolize beta-endorphin in response to a placebo challenge was described in "A study of placebo response," by L. Lasagna, F. Mosteller, J. M. von Felsinger and H. K. Beecher, *American Journal of Medicine*, vol. 16, 1954, pp. 770–79.

The Newcastle-upon-Tyne studies were published as two articles by Bernard E. Tomlinson, Garry Blessed, and Martin Roth: "Observations on the brains on non-demented old people," *Journal *of Neurological Science,* vol. 7, 1968, pp. 331–56; and "Observations on the brains of demented old people," *Journal of Neurological Science*, vol. 2, 1970, pp. 205–42.

3. MEMORY AND INTELLIGENCE: HOW MUCH IS LOST?

Samuel Johnson was quoted in *A Good Age* by Alex Comfort, New York: Simon and Schuster, 1976, p. 135; Comfort's own statement comes from the same book, pp. 10–11.

Robert Kahn's quotes come from interviews in the spring of 1974 and on May 19, 1979. His 1974 study is described in "Memory complaint and impairment in the aged: The effect of depression and altered brain function" (with Steven H. Zarit, Nancy M. Hilbert, and George Niederehe), *Archives of General Psychiatry*, vol. 32, Dec. 1975, pp. 1569–73. The article he wrote with Nancy Miller, "Adaptational factors in memory function in the aged," appeared in *Experimental Aging Research*, vol. 4, no. 4, 1978, pp. 273–89.

Jack Botwinick's statement on long-term memory is from his book, *Aging and Behavior* (2nd ed.), New York: Springer Publishing Company, 1978, p. 330.

The quote about tripping over forgotten objects was made by Donald Hebb, a prominent Canadian psychologist, in "On watching myself get old," *Psychology Today*, Nov. 1978, pp. 15–23.

Richard Besdine's statement about benign and malignant forgetfulness was made in an interview in Dec. 1977.

The two men answering the advertisement from the NYU medical center were interviewed at the clinic on June 14, 1979.

Lissy Jarvik's quote is from an interview on May 24, 1979, an idea on which she expanded in "Some thoughts on the psychobiology of aging," *American Psychologist*, vol. 30, 1975, pp. 576–83.

The Kahn and Miller quote is from their article, cited above.

Raymond T. Bartus describes his rhesus monkey work in "Aging in the rhesus monkey: Debilitating effects on short-term memory" (with Denise Fleming and H. R. Johnson), *Journal of Gerontology*, vol. 33, no. 6, 1978, pp. 858–71.

The story of Henry M., based on Brenda Milner's descriptions, is recounted in *Mechanics of the Mind* by Colin Blakemore, London: Cambridge University Press, 1977, pp. 93–96. Another excellent description appears in *Life Manipulation: From Test Tube Babies to Aging,* by David G. Lygre, New York: Walker and Company, 1979, p. 123. Milner herself described the patient in "Disorders of learning and memory after temporal lobe lesions in man," *Clinical Neurosurgery,* vol. 19, 1972, pp. 421–46. Henry's first quote is from the Lygre book, his second from Blakemore's.

Proof of the excitation of the hippocampus during periods of discovery is cited in *The Brain: The Last Frontier* by Richard M. Restak, Garden City, N.Y.: Doubleday & Company, 1979, p. 17.

A. T. Welford's quote about neural noise is from *Human Ageing,* Sheila M. Chown (ed.), Baltimore: Penguin Books, 1972, p. 97.

Robert Kastenbaum described his speeded task experiment in "Pre-experiencing age," *Psychology Today,* Dec. 1971, and in a series of interviews in 1978.

T. R. Anders' experiment is described in "The effects of age upon retrieval from short-term memory" (with J. L. Fozard and T. D. Lillyquist), *Developmental Psychology,* vol. 6, 1972, pp. 214–17.

Alex Comfort's index card analogy appears in *A Good Age,* cited above, p. 135.

Experiments on aging and memory are best summarized in *Aging and Behavior* by Jack Botwinick, cited above, pp. 311–63.

James Birren's quote appears in "Translations in gerontology— From lab to life: Psychophysiology and speed of response," *American Psychologist,* Nov. 1974, pp. 808–15.

Botwinick's quote comes from *Aging and Behavior,* cited above, p. 337.

David Schonfield describes his work in "Memory storage and age," *Nature,* vol. 28, 1965, p. 918, and "Memory storage and aging" (with E. A. Robertson), *Canadian Journal of Psychology,* vol. 20, 1966, pp. 228–36.

S. H. Davis and Walter Obrist describe their work in "Age differences in learning and retention of verbal material," *Cornell Journal of Social Relations,* vol. 1, 1966, pp. 95–103.

Paul Baltes and K. Warner Schaie's discussion of aging and intelligence appears in "Aging and I.Q.: The myth of the twilight years," *Psychology Today,* vol. 7, Mar. 1974, pp. 35–40.

The cohort factor and the value of longitudinal versus cross-sectional testing are discussed at length in Botwinick's *Aging and Behavior,* cited above, pp. 364–98.

Frances Wilkie and Carl Eisdorfer describe their work in "Intelligence and blood pressure in the aged," *Science*, vol. 172, 1971, pp. 959–62, as well as in a paper read at the Ninth International Congress of Gerontology in Kiev, U.S.S.R., in 1972.

Merrill Elias evaluates studies on blood pressure and intelligence, and describes his own research, in "The Influence of Essential Hypertension on Intellectual Performance: Causation or Speculation?" (with Michael A. Robbins and Norman Schultz), *Cardiovascular Disease, Aging and Behavior*, New York: Hemisphere Publishing/McGraw-Hill, 1985.

Kalidas Nandy describes his work with anti-brain antibodies in "Brain-reactive antibodies in aging and senile dementia," in *Alzheimer's Disease: Senile Dementia and Related Disorders*, Robert Katzman, Robert D. Terry, and Katherine L. Bick (eds.), New York: Raven Press, 1978, pp. 503–12; also in "Significance of brain-reactive antibodies in serum of aged mice," *Journal of Gerontology*, vol. 30, 1975, pp. 412–16; and in "Immune reactions in aging brain and senile dementia," in *The Aging Brain and Senile Dementia*, K. Nandy and I. Sherwin (eds), New York: Plenum Press, 1977, pp. 181–96.

Studies on hypodiploidy in the aged are described by Johannes Nielsen in "Chromosomes in senile dementia," *British Journal of Psychiatry*, vol. 115, 1968, pp. 303–09; and by Lissy F. Jarvik in "Organic brain syndrome and chromosome loss in aged twins," *Diseases of the Nervous System*, vol. 32, 1971, pp. 159–70.

Evidence for and against the terminal drop hypothesis is reviewed in "The terminal drop hypothesis: Fact or artifact?" by Ilene C. Siegler, *Experimental Aging Research*, vol. 1, no. 1, 1975, pp. 169–85. Among the most important studies in this area are R. W. Kleemeir, "Intellectual changes in the senium," *Proceedings of the American Statistical Association*, vol. 1, 1962, pp. 290–95; L. F. Jarvik and J. E. Blum, "Cognitive decline as predictor of mortality in twin pairs: A twenty-year-long study of aging," in *Prediction of Lifespan*, E. Palmore and F. C. Jeffers (eds.), Lexington, Mass.: D. C. Heath, 1971; and K. F. Riegel and R. M. Riegel, "Development, drop, and death," *Developmental Psychology,* vol. 6, no. 2, 1972, pp. 306–09.

M. A. Lieberman's quote is from "Psychological correlates of impending death: Some preliminary observations," *Journal of Gerontology*, vol. 20, 1965, pp. 492–97.

4. PSEUDOSENILITY

Richard Besdine's quotes are from an interview in Dec. 1977. Leslie Libow of Mount Sinai School of Medicine first coined the term "pseudosenility" in 1973 (see his article "Pseudosenility: Acute and reversible organic brain syndromes," *Journal of the American Geriatrics Society,* vol. 21, 1973, pp. 112–20). Before then, the term "psuedodementia" was used to refer to the mistaken diagnosis of depression as senility. Libow expanded the notion of a misdiagnosis of senility to include any reversible condition, not just depression, that produces senile symptoms and that is diagnosed as "senility" by a physician insufficiently attuned to ruling out those treatable causes.

Voltaire's aphorism was quoted in *Why Survive? Being Old in America* by Robert N. Butler, New York: Harper & Row, 1975, p. 200.

The Johns Hopkins study on adverse drug reactions is described in "Studies on the epidemiology of adverse drug reactions. III. Reactions in patients on a general medical service," L. G. Seidl, G. F. Thornton, J. W. Smith, and L. E. Cluff, *Bulletin of the Johns Hopkins Hospital*, vol. 119, 1966, pp. 299–315.

The study of adverse effects of hospitalization is described in "Complications in the care of 500 elderly hospitalized patients," by William Reichel, *Journal of the American Geriatrics Society*, vol. 13, 1965. pp. 973–81.

Robert E. Vestal of the Veterans Administration Hospital in Boise, Idaho, has written the most comprehensive and helpful summary of the problem of iatrogenic senility: "Drug use in the elderly: A review of problems and special considerations," *Drugs*, vol. 16, 1978, pp. 358–82. Vestal uses a somewhat more technical approach in his chapter, "Aging and pharmacokinetics: Impact of altered physiology in the elderly," in *Physiology and Cell Biology of Aging*, A. Cherkin et al. (eds.), New York: Raven Press, 1979.

Thomas Kalchthaler's statement was made during an interview on Dec. 22, 1977.

B. M. Learoyd describes his drug study in "Psychotropic drugs and the elderly patient," *Medical Journal of Australia*, vol. 1, 1972, pp. 1131–33.

Figures on drug expenditures by the aged in the United States come from R. M. Gibson, M. S. Mueller, and C. R. Fisher, "Age differences in health care spending, fiscal year 1976" *Social Security Bulletin*, vol. 40, 1977, pp. 3–14; the British figures are from K. O'Malley, T. G. Judge, and J. Crooks, "Geriatric clinical pharmacology and therapeutics," in Avery (ed.), *Drug Treatment,* Sydney: Adis Press; Edinburgh: Churchill Livingstone; Philadelphia: Lea & Febiger, 1976, pp. 123–42.

The New York study of drug-taking errors is described in "Medication errors made by elderly chronically ill patients," by D. Schwartz, M. Wang, L. Feitz, and M. E. W. Goss, *American Journal of Public Health*, vol. 52, 1962, pp. 2018–29.

The British study is described by D. M. Parkin, C. R. Henney, J. Quirk, and J. Crooks in "Deviation from prescribed drug treatment after discharge from hospital," *British Medical Journal*, vol. 2, 1976, pp. 686–88.

The figures on age-related changes in body water, body fat, and albumin levels, as well as Vestal's quote, are from his chapter in *Physiology and Cell Biology of Aging,* cited above.

Sheila Sherlock's work is described by S. Sherlock, A. G. Bearn, B. H. Billing, and J. C. S. Paterson, "Splanchnic blood flow in man by the bromsulfalein method: The relation of peripheral plasma bromsulfalein level to the calculated flow," *Journal of Laboratory and Clinical Medicine,* vol. 35, 1950, pp. 923–32.

Studies of age-related changes in antipyrine clearance are summarized in "Studies of drug disposition in the elderly using model compounds," by R. E. Vestal, A. J. J. Wood, R. A. Branch, G. W. Wilkinson, and D. G. Shand, in *Liver and Aging,* K. Kitani (ed.), New York and Amsterdam: Elsevier/North-Holland Biomedical Press, 1978.

Age-related changes in glomerular filtration rate are described in "The effect of age on creatinine clearance in man: A cross-sectional and longitudinal study," by J. W. Rose, R. Andres, J. D. Tobin, A. H. Norris, and N. W. Shock, *Journal of Gerontology*, vol. 31, 1976, pp. 155–63.

Vestal's quotes come from an interview on May 18, 1979, and from his review article "Drug use in the elderly," cited above.

Alexander Leaf's quote is from an interview on May 24, 1979.

Vestal's statement on multiple diseases is from his review article, cited above, p. 360. The statement that 85 percent of Americans over age sixty-five suffer from chronic illnesses comes from Butler's *Why Survive?* cited above, p. 175.

The National Center for Health Statistics survey was reported by Charles S. Wilder and Susan S. Jack, "Health characteristics of Persons 45 Years and Older," NCHS Working Paper Series, No. 19, March 1984, p. 12.

The figure on drug use per person was cited in "Research on aging burgeons as more Americans grow older" by Marsha F. Goldsmith, *JAMA* (Medical News), vol. 253, no. 10, March 8, 1985, p. 1375.

Kalchthaler's quote is from the 1977 interview.

William E. Thornton's description of the two middle-aged men appears in "Dementia induced by methyldopa with haloperidol," *New England Journal of Medicine*, vol. 294, 1976, p. 1222.

Vestal's comment was made in the 1979 interview.

Richard Mahler's quote is from "Differential diagnosis of impaired mental function in middle and late adult life. I. Medical diseases," *Proceedings of the Eisenhower Medical Center*, no. 1, spring 1975, p. 22.

The elderly woman with hypothyroidism is described by Knight Steel and Robert G. Feldman in "Diagnosing dementia and its treatable causes," *Geriatrics*, March 1979, pp. 79–88.

The North Carolina study of thyroid dysfunction is described in "Mental changes accompanying thyroid gland dysfunction," by P. C. Whybrow, A. J. Prange, and C. R. Treadway, *Archives of General Psychiatry*, vol. 20, Jan. 1979.

Mahler's comment is from *Proceedings of the Eisenhower Medical Center*, cited above, p. 23.

Ernest Gruenberg's statement is from an interview on Jan. 11, 1978.

Figures on suicide rates in the United States are from The National Center for Health Statistics, as cited in "Death by Choice" by Don Colburn, *The Washington Post,* Feb. 27, 1985, Health Section, p. 9.

Raymond Adams's quote is from "Examining for dementia at the bedside: Discussion," *Proceedings of the Eisenhower Medical Center,* vol. 1, spring 1975, pp. 20–21.

Robert N. Butler's quote appears in *Why Survive?* p. 230.

Ernest Gruenberg's comment is from the 1978 interview.

The case of Mrs. T. was recounted by Robert Kahn in an interview on May 19, 1979.

The National Institute on Aging quotes the rate of pseudosenility as 10 to 30 reversible conditions for every 100 cases of "dementia" in the aged.

Much of the information on the 100 or so reversible causes of "senility" is from a draft document, "Treatment possibilities for mental impairment in the elderly," distributed for comment by the National Institute on Aging in May 1979 and based on a conference on reversible dementia held in Bethesda, Md., on July 10–11, 1978. The draft appeared in final form as "Senility reconsidered," by Robert N. Butler, Richard Besdine, Jacob Brody, Leroy Duncan, Lissy Jarvik, and Leslie Libow, *Journal of the American Medical Association*, vol. 244, no. 3, 1980, pp. 259–63.

Knight Steel and Robert Feldman made their recommendations in "Diagnosing dementia and its treatable causes," cited above.

Robert Kahn's observations were made in the 1979 interview.

5. ALZHEIMER'S DISEASE: THE REAL SENILE DEMENTIA

Much of the information in this chapter is derived from *Alzheimer's disease: Senile Dementia and Related Disorders*, Robert Katzman, Robert D. Terry, and Katherine L. Bick (eds.), New York: Raven Press, 1978.

The mortality figures are from "Mortality of the aged with chronic brain syndrome. II," by Arthur Peck, Leon Wolloch, and Manual Rodstein, in Katzman, Terry, and Bick, *Alzheimer's Disease*, cited above, pp. 299–313.

The number of death certificates listing Alzheimer's disease is from the National Center for Health Statistics, Rockville, Md., "Vital statistics of the United States," 1976, cited by Robert N. Butler in his Alvin Goldfarb Memorial Lecture delivered in New York on May 4, 1978. The speech was reprinted as "Aging: Research leads and needs" in *Forum on Medicine*, Nov. 1979.

Figures on mortality from Alzheimer's disease are from "The prevalence and malignancy of Alzheimer's disease: A major killer" by Robert Katzman, *Archives of Neurology*, vol. 33, no. 4, 1976, pp. 217–18. The Swedish study on relative risk factors for Alzheimer's disease appears in "Senile dementia," by T. Larsson, T. Sjögren, and G. Jacobson, *Acta Psychiatria Scandinavia* (suppl. 167), vol. 39, 1963, pp. 3–259.)

Butler's quote is from his article "Aging: Research leads and needs," cited above.

The relatives of patients with Alzheimer's disease made their comments at a question-and-answer session sponsored by the Alzheimer's Disease Society (later known as the Alzheimer's Disease and Related Disorders Association), held in Hackensack, N.J., on June 12, 1979.

Eric Pfeiffer describes "early dementia" in "Clinical manifestations of senile dementia," in *Senile Dementia: A Biomedical Approach*, Kalidas Nandy (ed.), New York and Amsterdam: Elsevier/North-Holland Biomedical Press, 1978, p. 171.

Alois Alzheimer's landmark paper was "Uber eine eigenartige Erkrankung der Hirnrinde," *Zentrablbl. Nervenheilk.*, vol. 30, 1907, pp. 177–79.

The link between the autopsies of young soldiers killed in Korea and the realization that senility, like atherosclerosis, is not inevitable with age was suggested by Robert Butler in an interview on Dec. 28, 1977.

One early team to suggest the similarity between "pre-senile," and "senile" dementia was Meta Neumann and her husband, Robert Cohn, in their article, "Incidence of Alzheimer's disease in a large mental hospital: Relation to senile psychosis and psychosis with cerebral arteriosclerosis," *Archives of Neurology and Psychiatry,* vol. 69, 1953, pp. 615–36.

Jean Constantinidis reported his study of brain lesions in "Is Alzheimer's disease a major form of senile dementia? Clinical, anatomical, and genetic data," in Katzman, Terry, and Bick, *Alzheimer's disease*, cited above, pp. 15–25.

The Japanese study was reported by Haruo Matsuyama and Sadao Nakamura in "Senile changes in the brain in the Japanese: Incidence of Alzheimer's neurofibrillary change and senile plaque," in Katzman, Terry, and Bick, *Alzheimer's Disease*, cited above, pp. 287–97.

Information about plaques and tangles comes primarily from Robert Terry's chapter, "Physical changes of the aging brain," in *The Biology of Aging*, John A. Behnke, Caleb E. Finch, and Gairdner B. Moment (eds.), New York: Plenum Press, 1978, pp. 205–20, and from an interview with Terry on Dec. 21, 1977.

Denham Harman has described his free radical theory in a personal communication (1980), and in numerous publications, including "Free radical theory of aging: Nutritional implications," *Age*, vol. 1, Oct. 1978, pp. 145–52; "Free radical theory of aging:

Effect of dietary fat on central nervous system function" (with Shelton Hendricks, Dennis E. Eddy, and Jon Seibold), *Journal of the American Geriatrics Society*, vol. 24, no. 7, 1976, pp. 301–07; and "Free radical theory of aging: Inhibition of amyloidosis in mice by antioxidants; possible mechanism" (with Dennis E. Eddy and James Noffsinger), *Journal of the American Geriatrics Society*, vol. 24, no. 5, 1976, pp. 203–10.

Donald Crapper McLachlin describes his work with aluminum in "Aluminum and other metals in senile (Alzheimer) dementia" (with S. Karlik and U. DeBoni), in Katzman, Terry, and Bick, *Alzheimer's Disease*, cited above, pp. 471–85; also in "Aluminum, neurofibrillary degeneration and Alzheimer's disease" (with S. S. Krishnan and S. Quittkat), *Brain*, vol. 99, 1976, pp. 67–80; and "Aluminum-induced neurofibrillary degeneration, brain electrical activity and alterations in acquisition and retention" (with A. J. Dalton), *Physiological Behavior*, vol. 10, 1973, pp. 925–45.

D. Carleton Gajdusek describes his work with kuru, and its possible link to other forms of dementia, in "Transmissible virus dementia: The relation of transmissible spongiform encephalopathy to Creutzfeld-Jakob disease" (with Robert Traub and Clarence J. Gibbs, Jr.), in *Aging and Dementia*, W. Lynn Smith and Marcel Kinsbourne (eds.) New York: Spectrum Publications, 1977, pp. 91–172; and in "Subacute spongiform virus encephalophathies: The transmissible virus dementia" (with Clarence J. Gibbs, Jr.), in Katzman, Terry, and Bick, *Alzheimer's Disease,* cited above, pp. 559–75.

Robert Katzman's comment was made during the question-and-answer session of the Alzheimer's Disease Society, June 12, 1979.

Information about Gajdusek and Gibbs's most recent work was provided by Sylvia Shaffer, public information officer of the National Institute of Neurological and Communicative Disorders and Stroke.

Leonard Heston describes his work in "Genetic relationships in early onset Alzheimer's dementia" (with Mathew McGue and June White), *Annals of Internal Medicine*, in press; and in "Down's syndrome and Alzheimer's dementia: Defining an association," *Psychiatric Developments,* vol. 4, 1984, pp. 287–294.

Jean Constantinidis discusses the notion of inhibitor genes in his chapter "Is Alzheimer's disease a major form of senile dementia?", cited above.

The decline in acetylcholine levels in Alzheimer's disease was reported by Peter Davies, A. H. Verth, and A. J. F. Maloney, "Selective loss of central cholinergic neurons in Alzheimer's disease," *Lancet*, vol. 2, 1976, p. 1403; David Bowen, M. J. Goodhardt, A. J. Strong, C. B. Smith, P. White, N. M. Branston, L. Symon, and A. N. Davison, in *Brain Research*, vol. 117, 1976, pp. 503–07; and Elaine K. Perry, R. H. Perry, Garry Blessed, and Bernard E. Tomlinson, "Necroscopy evidence of central cholinergic deficits in senile dementia," *Lancet*, vol. 1, 1977, p. 189.

Peter Davies's quote is from "Research attempts to fight senility," by Harold M. Schmeck, Jr., New York *Times*, July 31, 1979, p. C-1.

Information on the diagnosis of Alzheimer's disease is derived from "Diagnosing dementia and its treatable causes," by Knight Steel and Robert G. Feldman, *Geriatrics*, Mar. 1979, pp. 79–88; "Diagnosis of senile and related forms of dementia," by Martin Roth, in Katzman, Terry, and Bick, *Alzheimer's Disease*, cited above, pp. 71–85; "Dementia in the elderly: Diagnosis and assessment," by Tom Arie, *British Medical Journal,* vol. 4, 1973, pp. 540–43; and in interviews with Robert Katzman on Dec. 21, 1977, and June 12, 1979, and Barry Reisberg on June 14, 1979.

A summary of PET, SPECT, and NMR appears in "Medical imaging" by Marvin B. Cohen, *Generations,* Winter 1984, pp. 37–40.

Katherine Bick's comment was made during an interview in 1979.

The quote from the daughter of an Alzheimer's patient is from the Alzheimer's Disease Society's 1979 question-and-answer session.

Eric Pfeiffer describes avoidance, confabulation, and perseveration in "Clinical manifestations of senile dementia," cited above, pp. 178–79.

Sir Martin Roth describes the aged violinist in "Diagnosis of senile and related forms of dementia," cited above. p. 77.

6. ALZHEIMER'S DISEASE: THE SCOTTS' STORY

This chapter is based on a weekend spent in Linda and Leonard Scott's home, Nov. 3–4, 1979, during which each member of the "Scott" family was interviewed at length. The professional opinions were garnered in interviews with Jack Friedman and Howard Hurtig on Nov. 5, 1979. Information for the epilogue came from an interview with Hurtig on May 6, 1985.

7. SENILITY "CURES": THE FAR OUT AND THE POSSIBLE

The Yeats quote is from his poem "The Tower," from *Selected Poems and Two Plays of William Butler Yeats*, M. L. Rosenthal (ed.), New York: The Macmillan Company/Collier Books, 1962, p. 96.

David A. Drachman describes his work in "Memory, dementia, and the cholinergic system," in *Alzheimer's Disease: Senile Dementia and Related Disorders*, Robert Katzman. Robert D. Terry, and Katherine L. Bick (eds.), New York: Raven Press, 1978, pp. 141–148. Peter Davies described his work in the same volume, "Studies on the neurochemistry of central cholinergic systems in Alzheimer's disease," pp. 453–59, and in an interview on Jan. 16, 1981. And Robert Harbaugh's experiment is described in "A slow death of the mind" by Matt Clark et al., *Newsweek,* Dec. 3, 1984, p. 62.

The NYU trials of Deanol and choline chloride are described in "Pharmacotherapy of senile dementia," by Barry Reisberg, Steven H. Ferris, and Samuel Gershon, a paper presented to the American Psychopathological Association, Mar. 1–2, 1979, in New York, and published in *Psychopathology in the Aged*, J. O. Cole (ed.), New York: Raven Press, 1980.

Other experiments with choline chloride are reported by W. D. Boyd, J. Graham White, G. Blackwood, I. Glen, and J. McQueen in *Lancet*, vol, 2, 1977, p. 711; and by R. C. Mohs, K. L. Cavis, J. R. Tinklenberg, L. E. Hollister, J. A. Yesavage, and B. S. Kopell, in the *American Journal of Psychiatry,* vol. 136, no. 10, 1979, pp. 1275–77.

Denham Harman describes his experiments with vitamin E in "Free radical theory of aging: Inhibition of amyloidosis in mice by antioxidants; possible mechanism" (with Dennis E. Eddy and James Noffsinger), *Journal of the American Geriatrics Society*, vol. 24, no. 5, 1976, pp. 203–10, and in a personal communication (June 26, 1974).

A. Hoffer's quotes are from "Senility and chronic malnutrition," *Journal of Orthomolecular Psychiatry*, vol. 3, no. 1, 1974, pp. 2–19.

James McConnell's experiment with flatworms is described in *Life Manipulation: From Test Tube Babies to Aging* by David G. Lygre, New York: Walker and Company, 1979, p. 124.

The quote from D. Ewen Cameron is from "The use of nucleic acid in aged patients with memory impairment," *American Journal of Psychiatry*, vol. 114, 1958, p. 943.

Augusto Britton's quote is from "Failure of ingestion of RNA to enhance human learning," by Augusto Britton, Leon L. Bernstein, Anthony J. Brunse, Matthew. W. Buttiglieri, Arthur Cherkin, John H. McCormack, and Donald J. Lewis, *Journal of Gerontology*, vol. 27, no. 4, 1972, pp. 478–81.

One trial of magnesium pemoline is described in "The effect of magnesium pemoline on cognition and behavior," by Carl Eisdorfer, James F. Conner, Frances L. Wilkie, *Journal of Gerontology*, vol. 23, 1968, pp. 283–88.

The warning about RNA in the gout-prone is from *Life Extension* by Durk Pearson and Sandy Shaw, New York: Warner Books, 1982, p. 170.

The caveat emptor for RNA products is from "Mind food," by Sandy Shakocius and Durk Pearson, *Omni,* May 1979, p. 57.

Ana Aslan's quote is from "Gerovital comes in from the cold," *Medical World News,* May 11, 1973, pp. 25–27. Descriptions of GH_3's action at the basic biological level are found in "That youth drug again: It seems to do something," *Medical World News*, Dec. 14, 1973, pp. 15–17; "A look at Gerovital—the 'youth' drug," by Saul Kent, *Geriatrics*, vol. 31, no. 12, 1976, pp. 95–102; and "The systematic use of procaine in the treatment of the elderly: A review," by Adrian Ostfeld, Cedric M. Smith, and Bernard A. Stotsky, *Journal of the American Geriatrics Society*, vol. 25, no. 1, 1977, pp. 1–19. A review of attempts to legalize the drug in the United States is in "Time marches on despite Gerovital," by Annabel Hecht, *FDA Consumer*, Mar. 1980, pp. 16–19.

The figures from California regarding Hydergine are mentioned in "Pharmacotherapy of senile dementia," by Reisberg, Ferris, and Gershon, cited above.

John R. Hughes's review appears in "An ergot alkaloid preparation (Hydergine) in the treatment of dementia: Critical review of the clinical literature" (with James G. Williams and Robert D. Currier), *Journal of the American Geriatrics Society*, vol. 24, no. 11, 1976. pp. 490–97.

The German study of Hydergine is described in "Long-term treatment of the symptoms of senile cerebral insufficiency: A prospective study of Hydergine," by J. Kugler, W. D. Oswald, U. Herzfeld, R. Seus, J. Pingel, and D. Welzel, *Dtsch. Med. Wschr.*, vol. 103, 1978, pp. 456–62.

Roland Branconnier and Jonathan Cole's quotes are from "The therapeutic efficacy of psychopharmacologic agents in senile organic brain syndrome," in *Senile Dementia: A Biomedical Approach*, Kalidas Nandy (ed.), New York and Amsterdam: Elsevier/North-Holland Biomedical Press, 1978, p. 273.

Martin Albert describes his work in "Subcortical dementia," in Katzman, Terry, and Bick, *Alzheimer's Disease*, cited above, pp. 173–80.

The trials of L-dopa at New York and Northwestern universities are described in "Pharmacotherapy of senile dementia" by Reisberg, Ferris, and Gershon, cited above. The two reports on L-dopa from the Royal Dundee Liff Hospital appear in "Trial of levodopa in senile dementia," by Christopher Lewis, Brian R. Ballinger, and Allan S. Presly, *British Medical Journal*, Mar. 4, 1978, p. 550; and "Levodopa in senile dementia" (letter), by Kate Johnson, Allan S. Presly, and Brian R. Ballinger, *British Medical Journal*, June 17, 1978, p. 1625.

Alfred Soffer's quote is from "Chelation therapy for arteriosclerosis," *Journal of the American Medical Association*, vol. 233, no. 11, 1975, p. 1206.

Branconnier and Cole's quote is from their chapter in Nandy's *Senile Dementia*, cited above, p. 281.

I. Zs.-Nagy describes his work and hypothesis in "Effects of centrophenoxine on the monovalent electrolyte contents of the large brain cortical cells of old rats," I. Zs.-Nagy, C. Pieri, C. Giuli, and M. Del Moro, *Gerontology*, vol. 25, no. 94, 1979, pp. 94–102.

Edward Schneider's comments are from "Life Extension" (with John D. Reed, Jr.), *The New England Journal of Medicine*, vol. 312, no. 18, May 2, 1985, p. 1162.

Information about the nootropics is from "Pharmacotherapy of senile dementia," by Reisberg, Ferris, and Gershon, cited above.

The original publication regarding hyperbaric oxygenation was "Hyperoxygenation effect on cognitive functioning in the aged,"

Eleanor A. Jacobs, Peter M. Winter, Harry J. Alvis, and S. Mouchly Small, *New England Journal of Medicine,* vol. 281, no. 14, 1969, pp. 753–57.

The Mount Sinai experiment with high-pressure oxygen is described in "Hyperbaric oxygen treatment of organic mental syndrome in aged persons," A. I. Goldfarb, N. J. Hochstadt, and J. H. Jacobson, *Journal of Gerontology,* vol. 27, 1972, pp. 212–17. The NIMH study was published as "The effects of hyperbaric and normobaric oxygen on cognitive impairment in the elderly," Allen Raskin, Samuel Gershon, Thomas H. Crook, Gregory Sathananthan, and Steven Ferris, *Archives of General Psychiatry,* vol. 35, Jan. 1978, pp. 50–56.

Normal pressure hydrocephalus was first described in "Symptomatic occult hydrocephalus with 'normal' cerebrospinal-fluid pressure: A treatable syndrome," R. D. Adams, C. M. Fisher, S. Hakim, R. G. Ojemann, and W. H. Sweet, *New England Journal of Medicine,* vol. 273, no. 3, 1965, pp. 117–26.

Howard Hurtig's comments are from an interview on Nov. 5, 1979.

Information about the Friendship Center is from "Reaching out to find and help 'mentally frail' elderly," by Janet S. Sainer, *Aging,* Nov.–Dec. 1974; "Components of a community based program for the frail elderly: Implications for adaptation and replication," by Janet S. Sainer, Sytske Ochs, Mary Levendos, and Donita Moorhus, presented to the Gerontological Society, annual meeting, Nov. 18–22, 1977, San Francisco; and an interview with Sytske Ochs of the Community Service Society of New York in Dec. 1977.

Reality orientation is described in "Reality orientation for the elderly mental patient," by James C. Folsom, *Journal of Geriatric Psychiatry*, vol. 2, no. 2, spring 1968, pp. 291–307; and "Reality orientation: A technique to rehabilitate elderly and brain-damaged patients with a moderate to severe degree of disorientation," by Louise P. Stephens, Washington, D. C.: American Psychiatric Association, 1975.

The SAGE program is described in "Senior Actualization and Growth Exploration (SAGE)" by Suzanne Fields, in *The New Old: Struggling for Decent Aging*, Ronald Gross, Beatrice Gross, and Sylvia Seidman (eds.), Garden City, N.Y.: Anchor Press/Doubleday, 1978, pp. 387–95.

8. MEDICAL AGEISM

Robert Butler told the anecdote about Morris Rocklin in an address on "Care of the aged: Perspectives on pain and discomfort" at the NIH Conference on Pain, Discomfort, and Humanitarian Care, Feb. 16, 1979, Bethesda, Md.

The story of "Mrs. Goode" is from an interview with Richard Shannon on Feb. 18, 1980.

Shura Saul's quote is from *Aging: An Album of People Growing Old*, New York: John Wiley & Sons, 1974.

Robert Butler's quote is from *Why Survive? Being Old in America*, New York: Harper & Row, 1975, p. 182.

Figures on old persons' utilization of medical care services are from R. M. Gibson and C. R. Fisher, "Age differences in health care spending, fiscal year 1977," *Social Security Bulletin*, vol. 41, 1979, pp. 2–16, and from Charles S. Wilder and Susan S. Jack, "Health characteristics of persons 45 years and older," NCHS Working Paper Series, No. 19, March 1984, p. 9.

Quotations from the Rand report are from "Geriatrics in the United States: Manpower projections and training considerations" by Robert L. Kane, David H. Solomon, John C. Beck, Emmett Keeler, and Rosalie A. Kane, Santa Monica, Calif.: Rand Corporation, 1980. A summary of the report is published in *New England Journal of Medicine*, vol. 302, no. 24, 1980, pp. 1327–32.

Donald Spence's quotes are from "Medical student attitudes toward the geriatric patient," by Donald L. Spence, Elliott M. Feigenbaum, Faith Fitzgerald, and Janet Roth, *Journal of the American Geriatrics Society*, vol. 16, no. 9, 1968, pp. 976–83.

Richard Shannon's quote is from the 1980 interview.

L. Thompson Bowles's quote is from an interview on Feb. 7, 1980.

Figures on the number of medical schools teaching geriatrics in 1976 and 1978 are from *Aging and Medical Education: Report of a Study*, Washington, D.C.: National Academy of Sciences, Institute of Medicine, Sept. 1978, pp. 38–39. Figures for 1981 are from "A study of geriatric training programs in the United States," by Alan S. Robbins, Susan Vivell, and John C. Beck, *Journal of Medical Education*, vol. 57, Feb. 1982, pp. 79–86.

The Kane group's quote is from "Geriatrics in the United States," cited above.

Robert Butler's quote is from *Why Survive?* cited above, p. 179.

L. Thompson Bowles's quote is from the 1980 interview.

Quotes from *The House of God* are from the book by Samuel Shem, New York: Dell Publishing Company, 1978, p. 38 and p. 13, respectively.

The quote from Donald Spence is from "Medical student attitudes toward the geriatric patient," cited above.

Patricia Blanchette's comments were made in an interview in June 1977, and appear in "Tomorrow's challenge: Health care for the elderly," by Robin Marantz Henig, *The New Physician*, vol. 26, no. 10, 1977, pp. 25–29.

Richard Shannon's quote is from the 1980 interview.

Robert Butler's quote is from an interview in June 1977, and appears in "Tomorrow's challenge: Health care for the elderly," cited above.

9. ENVIRONMENT: THE "SENILITY" REGULATOR

The story of Mary Larkin appears in "Alone: 8000 hidden elderly, confused, depressed, unfound by welfare," by LaBarbara Bowman, *The Washington Post,* Feb. 25, 1980, p. C–1.

The American Psychological Association's statement was reprinted in *Psychology of Adult Aging and Development*, Carl Eisdorfer and M. Powell Lawton (eds.), Washington, D.C.: American Psychological Association, 1973, pp. x–xi.

M. Powell Lawton states his Environmental Docility Hypothesis in "Sensory deprivation and the effect of the environment on management of the senile dementia patient," a paper presented at the National Institute of Mental Health Conference on Clinical Aspects of Alzheimer's Disease/Senile Dementia, Dec. 6–8, 1978, Bethesda, Md. p. 4.

Census data about the impoverished elderly are from *Statistical Abstracts of the United States,* U. S. Department of Commerce, Bureau of the Census, Washington, D.C.: Government Printing Office, 1981.

The University of Michigan experiment is described in "Toward an empathic model in architecture," L. A. Pastalan, Ann Arbor: Department of Architecture, University of Michigan, 1971.

Alex Comfort's quote is from *A Good Age*, New York: Simon and Schuster, 1976, p. 20.

The story about the ninety-year-old man was recounted by Max Henig on Apr. 20, 1979, on the occasion of his own ninetieth birthday.

Ernest Gruenberg's quotes are from an interview on Jan. 11, 1978.

A discussion of prosthetic environments is found in "Geriatric behavioral prosthetics" by Ogden R. Lindsley, in *New Thoughts on Old Age*, Robert Kastenbaum (ed.), New York: Springer Publishing Company, 1964, pp. 41–60.

M. Powell Lawton's quote is from "Sensory deprivation," cited above, p. 11.

The British nursing home study is described in "Status and spatial appropriation in eight homes for old people," by A. Lipman and R. Slater, *The Gerontologist*, vol. 17, 1977, pp. 250–55.

Advantages of furniture rearrangement in institutions is described in "Social interactions in geriatrics ward," by R. Sommer and H. Ross, *International Journal of Social Psychiatry*, vol. 4, 1958, pp. 128–33.

The benefits of a daily wine break are described in "Effects of wine on the interpersonal behavior of geriatric patients: An exploratory study," by Robert Kastenbaum and Philip E. Slater, in Kastenbaum's *New Thoughts on Old Age*, cited above, pp. 191–204.

M. Powell Lawton's quote is from "Sensory deprivation," cited above, p. 25.

The long-term-care wing at the Philadelphia Geriatric Center is described in "Evaluation: Designing for confused elderly people," by Bernard Liebowitz, M. Powell Lawton, and Arthur Waldman, *American Institute of Architects Journal*, Feb. 1979.

Western European approaches to housing the elderly are described in *Old People in Three Industrial Societies* by Ethel Shanas, Peter Townsend, Dorothy Wedderburn, Henning Friis, Poul Milhoj, and Jan Stehoewer, New York: Atherton Press, 1968: and *The Adult Years* by Wilbur Bradbury, New York: Time-Life Books, 1975. Another helpful comparative study is *The Honorable Elders: a Cross-Cultural Analysis of Aging in Japan*, by Erdman Palmore, Durham, N.C.: Duke University Press, 1975.

10. A LOOK TO THE FUTURE

Margaret Mead's quote is from an interview with Grace Hechinger, *Family Circle*, July 26, 1977.

Richard Kalish's quote is from "The new ageism and the failure models: A polemic," *The Gerontologist*, vol. 19, no. 4, 1979, pp. 398–402.

Gene Cohen's quote is from "Comment: Organic brain syndrome—reality orientation for critics of clinical interventions," *The Gerontologist*, vol. 18, no. 3, 1978, pp. 313–16.

Robert Butler's quote is from "Aging: Research leads and needs," *Forum on Medicine,* Nov. 1979, p. 724.

Figures on voting patterns in the elderly are from *Why Survive? Being Old in America,* by Robert N. Butler, New York: Harper & Row, 1975, p. 324.

A description of the politics of biomedical research funding, as applied to the growth of the National Cancer Institute, can be found in *Cancer Crusade: The Story of the National Cancer Act of 1971*, by Richard A. Rettig, Princeton, N.J.: Princeton University Press, 1977.

Bibliography

GENERAL REFERENCES

BOOKS

Binstock, Robert H., and Ethel Shanas (eds.). *Handbook of Aging and the Social Sciences.* New York: Van Nostrand Reinhold, 1976.

Birren, James E., and K. Warner Schaie (eds.). *Handbook of the Psychology of Aging.* New York: Van Nostrand Reinhold, 1977.

Botwinick, Jack. *Aging and Behavior.* 2nd ed.; New York: Springer Publishing Company, 1978.

Butler, Robert N. *Why Survive? Being Old in America.* New York: Harper & Row, 1975.

Chown, Sheila M. *Human Ageing.* Baltimore: Penguin Books, 1972.

Comfort, Alex. *A Good Age.* New York: Simon and Schuster, 1976.

Curtin, Sharon R. *Nobody Ever Died of Old Age.* Boston: Little, Brown, 1972.

Gross, Ronald, Beatrice Gross, and Sylvia Seidman (eds.). *The New Old: Struggling for Decent Aging.* Garden City, N.Y.: Anchor Press/Doubleday, 1978.

Jarvik, Lissy F. *Aging into the 21st Century: Middle-Agers Today.* New York: Gardner Press, 1978.

Lygre, David G. *Life Manipulation: From Test Tube Babies to Aging.* New York: Walker and Company, 1979.

Rosenfeld, Anne H. *New Views on Older Lives.* Rockville, Md.: National Institute of Mental Health, 1978.

283

Saul, Shura. *Aging: An Album of People Growing Old.* New York: John Wiley & Sons, 1974.

PERIODICALS

Baltes, Paul B., and K. Warner Schaie. "The myth of the twilight years," *Psychology Today*, Mar. 1974.

Clark, Matt, Mary Hager, and Dan Shapiro. "Epidemic of senility," *Newsweek*, Nov. 5, 1979, p. 95.

Diamond, Marian Cleeves. "The aging brain: Some enlightening and optimistic results," *American Scientist*, vol. 66, Jan.–Feb. 1978, pp. 66–71.

Greenberg, Joel. "Old age: What is normal?" *Science News*, vol. 115, Apr. 28, 1979, pp. 284–85.

Hebb, Donald O. "On watching myself get old," *Psychology Today*, Nov. 1978, pp. 15–23.

Henig, Robin Marantz. "Exposing the myth of senility," *The New York Times Magazine*, Dec. 3, 1978, pp. 156–67.

Schmeck, Harold M., Jr. "Research attempts to fight senility," *New York Times*, July 31, 1979, p. C-1.

SPECIAL REFERENCES

BOOKS

Cape, Ronald. *Aging: Its Complex Management.* Hagerstown, Md.: Harper & Row, 1978.

Frankfather, Dwight. *The Aged in the Community: Managing Senility and Deviance.* New York: Praeger, 1977.

Higbie, Les. *To Understand the Aging Process: The Baltimore Longitudinal Study of the National Institute on Aging.* Washington, D.C.: Department of Health, Education, and Welfare, 1978.

Katzman, Robert, Robert D. Terry, and Katherine L. Bick (eds). *Alzheimer's Disease: Senile Dementia and Related Disorders.* New York: Raven Press, 1978.

Nandy, Kalidas (ed.) *Senile Dementia: A Biomedical Approach.* New York and Amsterdam: Elsevier/North-Holland Biomedical Press, 1978.

Quarton, G. C., T. Melnechuk, and F. O. Schmitt. *The Neurosciences.* New York: Rockefeller University Press, 1967.

Smith, W. Lynn, and Marcel Kinsbourne (eds.) *Aging and Dementia.* New York: Spectrum Publications, 1977.

PERIODICALS

Alexander, D. A. " 'Senile dementia': A changing perspective," *British Journal of Psychiatry,* vol. 121, 1972, pp. 207–14.

Blum, June E., and Lissy F. Jarvik. "Intellectual performance of octogenarians as a function of education and initial ability," *Human Development,* vol. 17, 1974, pp. 364–75.

Butler, Robert N. "Aging: Research needs and leads," *Forum on Medicine,* Nov. 1979, pp. 716–25.

Jarvik, Lissy F. "Some thoughts on the psychobiology of aging," *American Psychologist,* vol. 30, 1975, pp. 576–83.

Plum, Fred. "Dementia: An approaching epidemic," *Nature,* vol. 279, May 1979, pp. 372–73.

Schwartz, Theodore B. "The specter of decrepitude," *New England Journal of Medicine,* vol. 299, no. 22, Nov. 30, 1978, pp. 1248–49.

Index

309

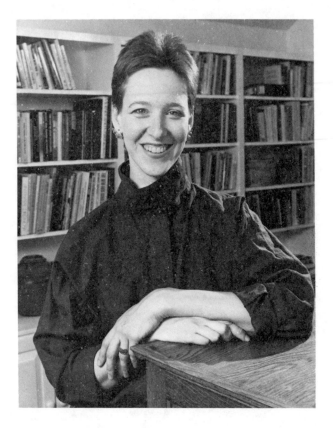

About the Author

ROBIN MARANTZ HENIG is a health and science writer whose work has appeared in *The New York Times Magazine*, *Woman's Day*, *The New Physician*, *Human Behavior*, and *BioScience*. Her previous books are *Your Premature Baby* and *How a Woman Ages*. Ms. Henig, who has a master's degree in journalism from Northwestern University, lives outside Washington, D.C., with her husband, Jeff, and their daughters, Jessica and Samantha.

AARP Books

ALONE—NOT LONELY, Independent Living for Women Over Fifty
by Jane Seskin
673-24814-3 $6.95

CAREGIVING, Helping An Aging Loved One
by Jo Horne
673-24822-4 $13.95

CATARACTS, The Complete Guide—from Diagnosis to Recovery—for Patients and Families
by Julius Shulman, M.D.
673-24824-0 $7.95

THE ESSENTIAL GUIDE TO WILLS, ESTATES, TRUSTS, AND DEATH TAXES
by Alex J. Soled
673-24809-7 $12.95

FITNESS FOR LIFE, Exercises for People Over 50
by Theodore Berland
673-24812-7 $12.95

THE GADGET BOOK, Ingenious Devices for Easier Living
Edited by Dennis R. La Buda
673-24819-4 $10.95

IT'S YOUR CHOICE, The Practical Guide to Planning a Funeral
by Thomas C. Nelson
673-24804-6 $4.95

KEEPING OUT OF CRIME'S WAY, The Practical Guide for People Over 50
by J. E. Persico with George Sunderland
673-24801-1 $6.95

LIFE AFTER WORK, Planning It, Living It, Loving It
by Allan Fromme
673-24821-6 $6.95

LOOKING AHEAD, How to Plan Your Successful Retirement
673-24829-1 $9.95

MEDICAL AND HEALTH GUIDE FOR PEOPLE OVER FIFTY
by Dartmouth Institute for Better Health
673-24816-X $14.95

THE MYTH OF SENILITY, The Truth About the Brain and Aging
by Robin Marantz Henig
673-24831-3 $14.95

**NATIONAL CONTINUING CARE DIRECTORY, Retirement
Communities with Prepaid Medical Plans**
Edited by Ann Trueblood Raper
673-24813-5 $13.95

THE OVER EASY FOOT CARE BOOK
by Timothy P. Shea, D.P.M., and Joan K. Smith
673-24807-0 $6.95

PLANNING YOUR RETIREMENT HOUSING
by Michael Sumichrast, Ronald G. Shafer, and Marika Sumichrast
673-24810-0 $8.95

**POLICY WISE, The Practical Guide to Insurance Decisions for
Older Consumers**
by Nancy H. Chasen
673-24806-2 $5.95

SUNBELT RETIREMENT
by Peter A. Dickinson
673-24832-1 $11.95

**SURVIVAL HANDBOOK FOR WIDOWS (and for relatives and
friends who want to understand)**
by Ruth J. Loewinsohn
673-24820-8 $5.95

TRAVEL EASY, The Practical Guide for People Over Fifty
by Rosalind Massow
673-24817-8 $8.95

**WHAT TO DO WITH WHAT YOU'VE GOT, The Practical Guide
to Money Management in Retirement**
by Peter Weaver and Annette Buchanan
673-24805-4 $7.95

YOUR VITAL PAPERS LOGBOOK
673-24833-X $4.95

For complete information write: AARP Books, 1900 East Lake
Avenue, Glenview, IL 60025 or contact your local bookstore.

Prices subject to change.

Scott, Foresman and the American Association of Retired Persons have joined together to bring you *Information You Can Count On!*

800. **What to Do with What You've Got:** The Practical Guide to Money Management in Retirement. *$7.95/AARP member price $5.80.*

801. **Planning Your Retirement Housing.** *$8.95/AARP member price $6.50.*

803. **Policy Wise:** The Practical Guide to Insurance Decisions for Older Consumers. *$5.95/AARP member price $4.35.*

804. **It's Your Choice:** The Practical Guide to Planning a Funeral. *$4.95/AARP member price $3.00.*

805. **The Essential Guide to Wills, Estates, Trusts and Death Taxes.** *$12.95/AARP member price $9.45.*

806. **The Over Easy Foot Care Book.** *$6.95/AARP member price $4.95.*

807. **National Continuing Care Directory:** Retirement Communities with Prepaid Medical Plans. *$13.95/AARP member price $9.95.*

808. **Survival Handbook for Widows** (and for relatives and friends who want to understand). *$5.95/AARP member price $4.35.*

809. **Life After Work:** Planning It, Living It, Loving It. *$6.95/AARP member price $4.95.*

Join AARP today and enjoy valuable benefits

Join the American Association of Retired Persons, the national organization which helps people like you, age 50 and over, realize their full potential in so many ways!

The rewards you'll reap with AARP will be many times greater than your low membership dues. And your membership also includes your spouse!

Your AARP benefits

- Modern Maturity magazine
- Legislative work benefiting mature persons
- Nonprofit Pharmacy Service
- Quality Group Health Insurance
- Specially priced Motoring Plan
- Community Volunteer Activities
- Hotel & Car Rental Discounts
- Travel Service
- Tax-Aide Program to help with your taxes

60% of dues is designated for Association publications. Dues outside continental U.S.: $7 one year, $18 three years. Please allow 3 to 6 weeks for receipt of membership kit.

☐ one year/$5
☐ three years/$12.50 (saves $2.50)   LHAA
☐ ten years/$35 (saves $15)
☐ Check or money order enclosed, payable to AARP. DO NOT SEND CASH
☐ Please bill me.

Name (please print)

Address   Apt.

City

State   Zip

Date of
Birth _____ mo/_____ day/_____ year

☐ *Start my membership in NRTA (a division for those in or retired from education)*   LHNA

Information You Can Count On!

810. **Alone - Not Lonely:** Independent Living for Women Over Fifty. *$6.95/AARP member price $4.95*

811. **Travel Easy:** The Practical Guide for People Over 50. *$8.95/AARP member price $6.50*

812. **Keeping Out of Crime's Way:** The Practical Guide for People Over 50. *$6.95/AARP member price $4.95*

815. **Cataracts:** The Complete Guide From Diagnosis to Recovery for Patients and Families. *$7.95/AARP member price $5.80*

817. **Looking Ahead:** How to Plan Your Successful Retirement. *$9.95/AARP member price $6.95*

181. **Your Vital Papers Logbook:** *$4.95/AARP member price $2.95*

HOW TO ORDER

To order state book name and number, quantity and price (AARP members: be sure to include your membership no. for discount) and add $1.75 *per order* for shipping and handling. *All orders must be prepaid.* For your convenience we accept checks, money orders, VISA and MasterCard (credit card orders must include card no., exp. date and cardholder signature). *Please allow 4 weeks for delivery.*

Send your order today to:
AARP Books, Scott, Foresman and Co., 400 S. Edward St., Mt. Prospect, IL 60056

AARP Books are co-published by AARP and Scott, Foresman and Co., sold by Scott, Foresman and Co., and distributed to bookstores by Farrar, Straus and Giroux.

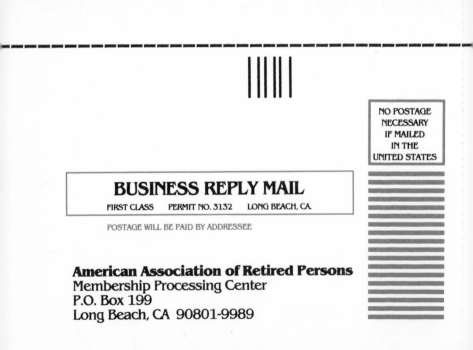

NO POSTAGE
NECESSARY
IF MAILED
IN THE
UNITED STATES

BUSINESS REPLY MAIL

FIRST CLASS   PERMIT NO. 3132   LONG BEACH, CA.

POSTAGE WILL BE PAID BY ADDRESSEE

American Association of Retired Persons
Membership Processing Center
P.O. Box 199
Long Beach, CA 90801-9989

Information You Can Count On!

810. **Alone - Not Lonely:** Independent Living for Women Over Fifty.
$6.95/*AARP member price $4.95*

811. **Travel Easy:** The Practical Guide for People Over 50. $8.95/*AARP
member price $6.50*

812. **Keeping Out of Crime's Way:** The Practical Guide for People Over 50.
$6.95/*AARP member price $4.95*

815. **Cataracts:** The Complete Guide From Diagnosis to Recovery for Patients
and Families. $7.95/*AARP member price $5.80*

817. **Looking Ahead:** How to Plan Your Successful Retirement.
$9.95/*AARP member price $6.95*

181. **Your Vital Papers Logbook:** $4.95/*AARP member price $2.95*

HOW TO ORDER

To order state book name and number, quantity and price (AARP members: be sure to
include your membership no. for discount) and add $1.75 *per order* for shipping and
handling. *All orders must be prepaid.* For your convenience we accept checks, money
orders, VISA and MasterCard (credit card orders must include card no., exp. date and
cardholder signature). *Please allow 4 weeks for delivery.*

Send your order today to:
**AARP Books, Scott, Foresman and Co., 400 S. Edward St.,
Mt. Prospect, IL 60056**

AARP Books are co-published by AARP and Scott, Foresman and Co., sold by Scott,
Foresman and Co., and distributed to bookstores by Farrar, Straus and Giroux.

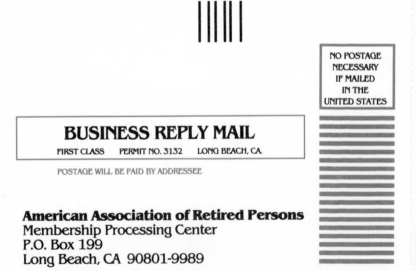

NO POSTAGE
NECESSARY
IF MAILED
IN THE
UNITED STATES

BUSINESS REPLY MAIL

FIRST CLASS   PERMIT NO. 3132   LONG BEACH, CA.

POSTAGE WILL BE PAID BY ADDRESSEE

American Association of Retired Persons
Membership Processing Center
P.O. Box 199
Long Beach, CA 90801-9989